Hollywood's Hottest Actresses Love Kate Somerville!

"Whenever my skin looks youthful and glowey, I thank God, my mom, and Kate Somerville. I don't know what I would do without her and them."

— Julia Louis-Dreyfus

"Kate has completely transformed my skin. For the first time in my life, at age 40, I'm getting compliments on how beautiful my skin is. I think that says it all."

— Debra Messing

"Kate Somerville has literally changed the face of skin care, from the inside out. Thanks to Kate, my skin always looks great!"

— Kate Walsh

"Kate has made me feel so good about my skin. She's changed it to the best it's ever been, and her skin care is by far the best I've ever used! I adore her and think she is a genius."

— Lisa Rinna

"I ran into an actress at Starbucks. She looked at least 20 years younger than the last time I saw her. She looked amazing. When I asked her why she looked so good, she answered, 'I switched from drinking coffee to drinking tea.' She smiled. I didn't believe her. A few weeks later I ran into her at Kate Somerville . . . I knew it was more than the tea."

— Jennifer Coolidge

Complexion Perfection!

Complexion Perfection!

Your Ultimate Guide to Beautiful Skin
by Hollywood's Leading Skin Health Expert

Kate Somerville

HAY HOUSE, INC.
Carlsbad, California • New York City
London • Sydney • Johannesburg
Vancouver • Hong Kong • New Delhi

Published and distributed in the United States by: Hay House, Inc.: www.hayhouse.com • *Published and distributed in Australia by:* Hay House Australia Pty. Ltd.: www.hayhouse.com.au • *Published and distributed in the United Kingdom by:* Hay House UK, Ltd.: www.hayhouse.co.uk • *Published and distributed in the Republic of South Africa by:* Hay House SA (Pty), Ltd.: www.hayhouse.co.za • *Distributed in Canada by:* Raincoast: www.raincoast .com • *Published in India by:* Hay House Publishers India: www.hayhouse.co.in

Design: Amy Gingery   •   *Photography by:* Jim Jordan and Jeff Xander

Library of Congress Cataloging-in-Publication Data

Somerville, Kate.
   Complexion perfection! : your ultimate guide to beautiful skin by Hollywood's leading skin health expert / Kate Somerville. -- 1st ed.
       p. cm.
   ISBN 978-1-4019-2462-1 (hardcover : alk. paper) -- ISBN 978-1-4019-2463-8 (Tradepaper : alk. paper)   1. Skin--Care and hygiene. I. Title.
   RL87.S66 2010
   646.7'2--dc22
                                        2009024198

ISBN: 978-1-4019-2462-1

13   12   11   10   4   3   2   1
1st edition, March 2010

Printed in China

This book is dedicated to all of the inspirational women in my life. To my clients, friends, and family. To those I have cared for and who have cared for me. To each woman who has trusted, supported, and loved me unconditionally. Because of all of you, my dreams, and this book, have been made possible.

Contents

PART III: Complexion Transformation!

Client Transformations: Joanna Crane • Tracy Pitera • Karina Macias • Glen O'Connor Michelle Huang • Fay McCallister • Jim Row • Jenna Zickerman • Linda Cooper Carola Gonzales • Shayne • Jean Liu • Arla Jordan • Lori Lerner • Cathi Myers

PART IV: Complexion Affection!

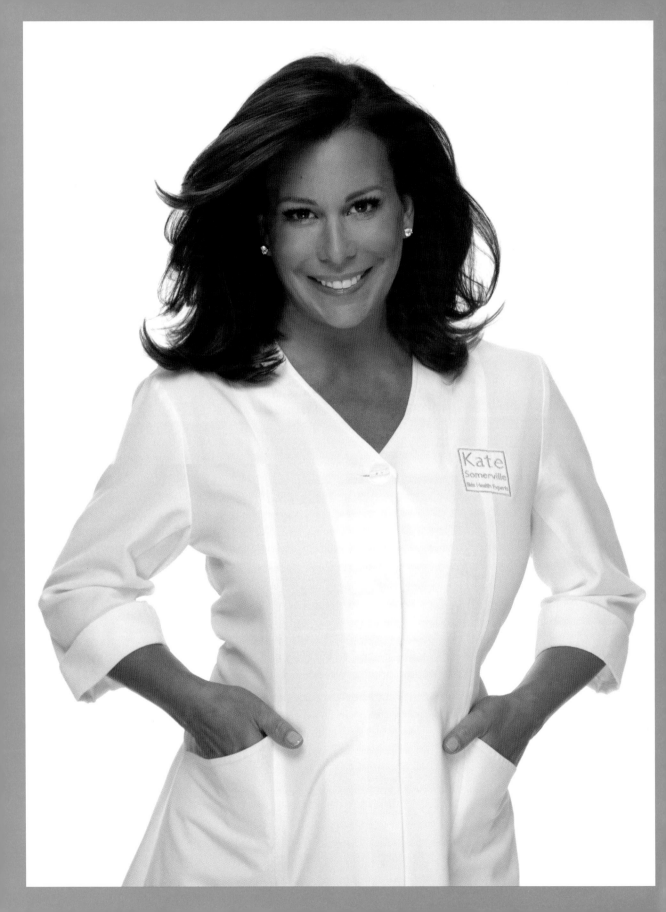

Preface

I am a paramedical esthetician, also
known as a clinical facialist, and have been
practicing for almost 20 years. As a
specialized facialist, I've spent most of my professional life
working side by side with dermatologists and cosmetic surgeons,
complementing their treatment strategies, with a focus on improving
skin health. Twenty years, five days a week, eight hours a day, is a lot
of time spent caring for skin! That's almost 50,000 hours. Wow—that
even surprises *me*. Skin care is more to me than just a job—
it's honestly my calling.

Over the years, I've seen so many people who were overcome with grief because of their skin challenges. They were all searching for one simple thing: a healthy complexion. I can't tell you how many clients have cried in my chair because they were distraught and feeling powerless. I've watched these men and women struggle with the state of their skin, and it's heartbreaking. Whether it's the emotional turmoil caused by acne or the anxiety associated with aging, insecurities can negatively influence how these individuals see themselves, how others see them, and how they live their lives.

This book is for every woman and man who wants—*yearns* for—gorgeous, glowing skin. Healthy skin is not a sign of vanity or privilege; healthy skin is every person's *right*. Whether you've never had it or you want to get it back, it's my professional goal to make radiant skin your reality. Whether you look tired and run-down, are plagued by breakouts, or are showing the signs of aging, this book is designed to give you the information and motivation you need to get your skin—and your spirit—in shape.

You may be like the many clients who have come to me after trying everything. They've spent hundreds (even thousands!) of dollars, tried a multitude of products, and popped controversial pills, yet they haven't seen results; or worse, they've experienced damaging side effects. I understand the frustration. There's so much out there. Just stepping into the cosmetics department of any retailer is enough to cause anxiety and confusion. What treatments to choose? What supplements to take? What ingredients to look for? What products to buy? The "what?" list goes on and on.

So I sit with my clients and tune in to their skin and their stories, because beauty is more than skin-deep. I dig. I learn about their lives, their families, and their challenges—complexion oriented and beyond. I know when they're head over heels in love or simply in over their heads. How? Sometimes they tell me, but mostly I know because the glow is either there or it's not.

Our skin is a reflection of our deepest selves. The expression "It's written all over your face" is so true. We absolutely wear our lives on our faces: our joys and pains, our loves and losses, our victories and surrenders. Our skin speaks of our present, tells tales of our past, and foreshadows our future. So, while some people read the lines on palms, I read the lines on faces.

Haven't you looked in the mirror during a challenging time and witnessed its undeniable mark on your face: dark circles, puffy eyes, furrowed brow? I certainly have. I've battled my own complexion chaos my entire life. I've had eczema since I was a child. To this day, when I'm traveling; not eating right; drinking too much caffeine; or not stopping to breathe, smile, and let go, my eczema comes back with a vengeance. It's a not-so-subtle message telling me to slow down. I look tired, my skin is lifeless, and, let's be honest, I look older. I need a "skin-tervention"! That can mean taking a hike with the dog, relaxing in a long bath, squeezing some fresh juice, getting a facial, or spending time with my husband. And remembering to just breathe . . .

I've spent years working on myself and my soul. Yet I only recently came to understand how effective this work can be in healing the human body and our skin. The state of our skin reflects the present state of our being. Since it's the largest organ that's visible to the eye, our skin is a reflection of what's going on in our heads and our hearts. I strongly believe in technology, advances in science, and the latest and greatest ingredients; after all, I use them in my clinic and in my product collection. But they're only a few tools in my workshop, or one dimension of total skin wellness. Healthy, radiant skin is the result of a healthy, radiant spirit, body, and mind. Balance is the foundation—and it's something that I'm still learning to practice myself. Like you, I have a lot of responsibilities. I'm a mom, the CEO of a successful business, a wife, a friend, and a daughter. And like you, my time and energy are often limited.

This guide isn't meant to overwhelm you, but rather to inspire you toward your absolute best. So in these pages, I break down for you what I've been breaking down for my clients for years. I want you to reach new heights with your skin and with your life. *You can do it!* It's not too early and, I promise you, it's not too late. I'm almost 40, but my skin looks better now than it did when I was 20, thanks to what I've learned and applied over the years.

I'll share my multidimensional approach to skin care with you, talk about diet and its effect on your complexion, and uncover the role your mind and spirit play with regard to your skin. I'll explain what's out there in terms of treatments and products, what I believe in, and what I've seen work and how. I'll show you some incredible skin makeovers, which use my philosophy and the very tools outlined in this book. The motto at my clinic is "Changing skin, changing lives." It might seem dramatic, but you'll find that healthy skin gives you the confidence to meet any challenge with strength.

I read an interview with Michelle Obama in *Oprah* magazine, and she said her happiness was directly tied to how she felt about herself. I think most of us are like this—when we feel good about ourselves, we are stronger and meet the world better. I know that when my skin looks healthy, glowing, and clear, I feel better about myself. How I feel influences the decisions I make and the way I care for my friends, my business, and my family.

Everyone has a right to that radiance; it's not just reserved for celebrities, brides-to-be, or those who are simply born that way. You're in control. You have the power to change your skin and change your life. It's more than possible. I see skin change every day, whether it's breakouts vanishing, full-blown rosacea clearing up, or the lines of aging diminishing. I'm passionate about the partnership with my clients and with those I share advice. Now I want *you* to have skin you're proud of. It's my job to provide you with the knowledge and motivation to do it; it's *your* job to bring the trust and commitment.

I've divided the book into four sections. In Parts I and II, I give you the information and tools you need to change your skin. In Part III, I apply that to 15 skin makeovers on real clients so that you can see the results of the strategy applied. And finally, in Part IV, we explore affectionate ways to further enhance your complexion by getting professional hair, makeup, and fashion advice from friends I call "my Hollywood Glam Squad."

I promise you, the path to complexion perfection is just around the corner. Let's get started!

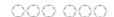

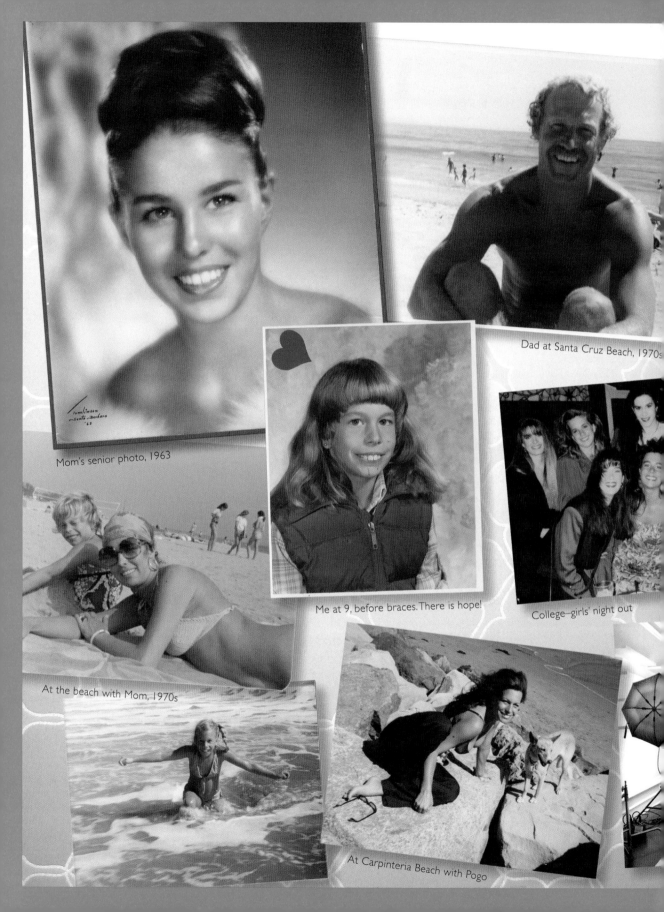

Mom's senior photo, 1963

Dad at Santa Cruz Beach, 1970s

Me at 9, before braces. There is hope!

College—girls' night out

At the beach with Mom, 1970s

At Carpinteria Beach with Pogo

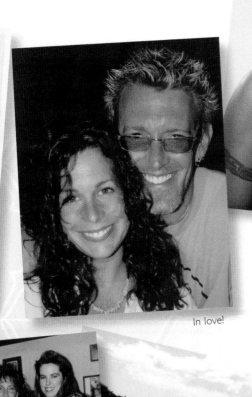

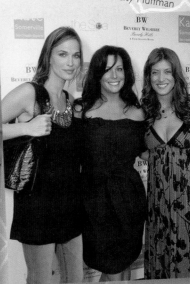

My family: Landa and Chae and me

In love!

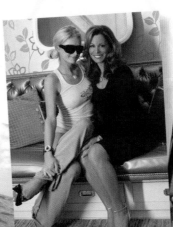

People magazine shoot with Paris Hilton

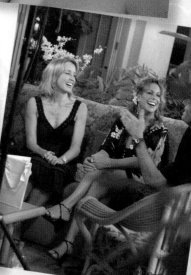

Maui press event with Felicity Huffman

My son and me in Hawaii

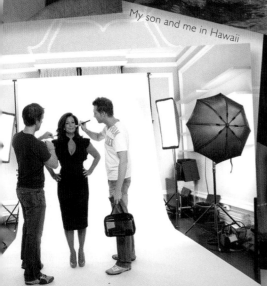

It takes a village!

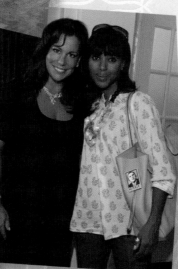

Emmy event with Kerry Washington

Press event with Molly Sims and Kate Walsh

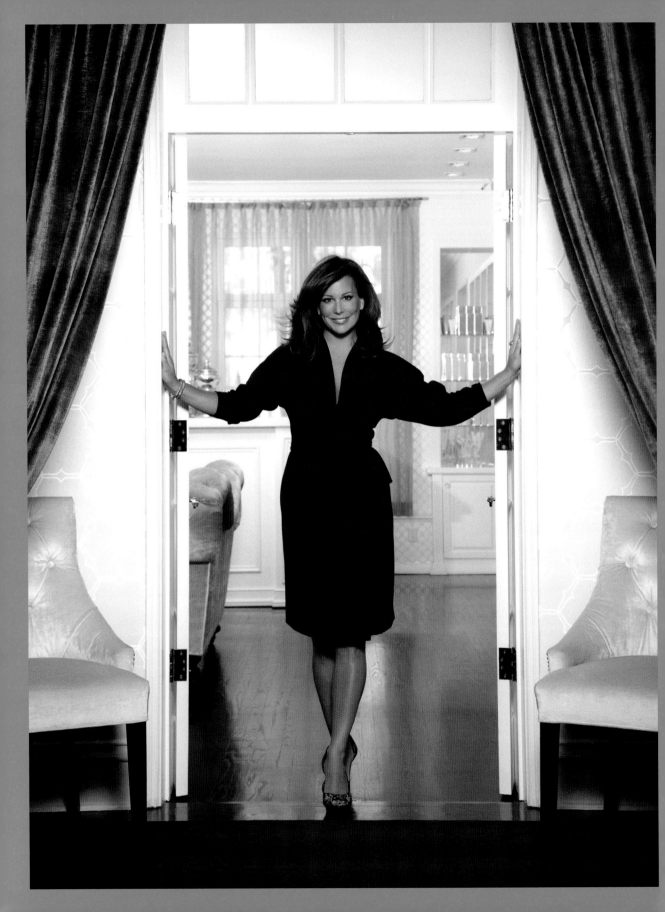

How I Became the "Guru of Glow"

I was born in central California to two creative and loving parents, both blessed with good looks and charisma. My mother was the head cheerleader at California State University, Fresno, and my father was the star football player. They were so much fun and full of life; everyone adored them. Just after college, they married and became teachers: my dad was a football coach and physical-education teacher, while my mom was a continuation teacher for rebellious youth. My mom was always able to connect with those who were lost, and my father was a strong leader. Both had huge hearts and were incredibly kind.

When I was a child living in Fresno, life seemed perfect. Being teachers, my parents would be in school when I was, and then we spent our afternoons together at home. Later, we moved to the foothills of the Sierra Nevada mountains, where my parents bought a beautiful piece of land and planned to build a house. In the meantime, we lived in a huge barn on the property, and my mom designed the whole space on her own. I loved this time of my life and remember it affectionately. But things did begin to change.

This was the '70s, and it was all about sex, drugs, and rock 'n' roll. The fun that filled my parents' early years started to take over. The party lifestyle soon ruled my mom, and she and my dad began to fight nonstop. The situation escalated as her drug and alcohol dependencies grew. She just couldn't be a mom anymore . . . or a wife, for that matter. Just around the time we broke ground for our new home, she left us and went to live in Santa Barbara. I was nine years old and can clearly remember the feelings I had—it was so painful. I knew she loved me, but I didn't know what I could do to make her come back. In many ways I was relieved she was gone, since the fighting stopped. But it was the worst feeling in the world to be a young girl without a mom.

For the next year it was just my dad and me, living in the barn on our land. It was incredibly eclectic and artistic, with a beautiful garden, a trailer for a kitchen, and an outhouse for a bathroom! I was the only person I knew who lived this way, and I'm convinced it was a source of my creativity. We'd always have family friends over, and every weekend seemed like a celebration.

It seems funny that I grew up to be in the beauty world, because I was such a tomboy in those days. I'd ride my horse, Ginger, to the school bus stop every day. When the bus came, I'd let her go, and she'd run straight back home. In the afternoon, I'd walk the two miles home, giving me a lot of time to daydream. So even though I missed my mother, the chaos had stopped and life was pretty good.

I'd visit my mom in Santa Barbara for a few days at a time, but she was very unstable. As a kid, I didn't totally understand what was going on, but I did feel the turmoil. Sometimes I'd be at home with my dad, and my mom would call in a depressed state, usually under the influence of drugs or alcohol. It got to where she became unrecognizable. I was so young and felt powerless . . . and here's where my skin troubles began. The chaos I felt inside showed up outside. I developed hives *everywhere:* on my palms, on the soles of my feet, between my toes, and on my eyelids. My emotional distress was channeled into this severe rash that flared up without warning. I felt responsible for my mom, but I was just a kid. There was nothing I could do, for her *or* my hives. I tried soaking in baths; applying gels, lotions, and creams; taking medication; anything and everything. But nothing worked. I was a mess, and no amount of baths, pills, or potions could fix what was going on inside.

My father was dealing with his own stuff—my mom leaving and his new role as a single parent. He remarried soon after my parents split, and his new wife had her own kids who were around my age. It was a major adjustment for me as it is with many children in blended families. I was vulnerable without my mom, and my father's new marriage brought additional challenges. Things at home were not easy and life felt like a constant struggle.

About this time, I broke out with eczema from head to toe. There were patches on my hands, my arms, my scalp, and my face. My skin would get so dry and inflamed it would crack and bleed. If you've ever experienced a severe case of eczema, then you know how uncomfortable it can be. I was overwhelmed by pain, both physical and mental. Doctors prescribed creams that supressed the awful itching, but the creams never cured the wounds. I felt so uncomfortable in my own skin, literally and figuratively. And it's taken my entire life to find physical *and* emotional comfort for myself.

Things were such a mess at home that when I was 15, my dad sent me to see a counselor. There are good counselors and bad ones, and this was a good one who gave me powerful advice. She said to me, "Katie, I can't believe what I'm about to say to you, but you need to leave and find a home better suited to what you need. You're struggling there too much. You need to survive and you need to thrive. Let's figure out how to get you there." So with her blessing I left home and moved in with my best friend and her family. While moving out was the best thing I could have done for myself, it created a sense of homelessness and isolation that took years to overcome. The truth is, until about five years ago, I felt like a visitor everywhere I went.

Since I didn't have much guidance, I started to make poor choices in my teens, but by the time I was 18, I'd straightened out and decided to go to college. I went to Fresno State to pursue a degree in design and began dating a great guy. I also met an individual who would ultimately become the most influential woman in my life—my boyfriend's mother, Barbara Wells.

Barbara was truly amazing; she understood everything I was going through. One day she held me in her arms and said, "I want you to know I'm here for you, and I love you unconditionally. You've never had someone show you unconditional love." She held on to me and said, "Cry." It was the most healing moment in my life.

I would go on and on to Barbara about my troubles and my disappointments. And then one time she told me, "You know, you have a choice. You can make your life good or you can continue to dwell on your hardships." I honestly didn't know that I had a choice.

Barbara Wells was loving and supportive, and she taught me that I didn't have to live in chaos. I was in control of my life, and I had the power to change whatever it was I didn't like. I could get things under control and be whatever I wanted to be, have whatever I wanted to have, and achieve whatever I wanted to achieve. Even today I continue to replay her words of encouragement in my head. Barbara was my guiding light, showing me that anything is possible in life. (I apply this to skin, too—we can turn it around!) After having battled cancer for ten years, she died from the disease when I was about 20. Nevertheless, she remains the most inspirational woman I have ever known. Her message continues to guide me, personally and professionally.

Because of Barbara, I was finally able to make decisions based on what I wanted. I had always wanted to live in the coastal town of Cambria and I made the decision to move there. None of my friends believed I'd do it. But I did— I picked up and went!

I had no money, but there I was in my little blue Volkswagen Bug on the two-lane highway to Cambria, one of the most beautiful towns on Earth. And that's where and when my life started to change. I got three waitressing jobs and worked hard. I've always had a strong work ethic, which I get from my dad. He's a rancher now—a cowboy, really—who raises cattle. His way is if you fall down, then get up, dust yourself off, and get going.

I didn't tell my mother I was in Cambria because I needed to be away from her situation; it was just too painful. I had to get myself off the ground and work on letting go of my childhood struggles. I lived with my boyfriend at the time in a cottage close to the beach, and it was in that beachside bungalow that I began to heal—and so did my eczema. For the first time, I got a handle on it. It no longer controlled my life! The awful dryness and rashes disappeared in most areas and rarely flared up. I ate well, lived healthily, and could focus on the present, not the past. And in that healthy space, with an emerging sense of self and strength, I began to find direction.

In Fresno, I'd made a really good friend who was a dermatologist. She and I would talk endlessly about my eczema and all of the effort I'd put into healing myself. I knew that I didn't always want to be a waitress, so she suggested I get a degree in esthetics.

At the time, the field of esthetics was very new. Yet I was always intrigued by skin health and beauty, and this seemed like something I could finally sink my teeth into. So I went back to school, and a few months later I had my California esthetician license. It's a fairly simple qualification to get and, truthfully, does not adequately prepare you for all of the skin conditions you encounter or available solutions.

While I was in school, I had an idea. I knew I wanted to work side by side with doctors, to complement their services. This was unusual at the time, as most estheticians were facialists employed by spas. So I put together a business plan, and shortly after graduation opened my own clinic inside a cosmetic surgeon's office south of Cambria, in San Luis Obispo. I didn't know anything about running a business and was scared to death! But I overcame my fear and just did it. I was like a sponge, absorbing all that I could in the process. I learned everything I could about skin care, observed surgeries, and was fascinated by what was possible. I met other estheticians and nurses who were working with doctors, as I was. This was the very beginning of a burgeoning field.

It was now the '90s, and there were lots of advances taking place in skin care and technology. It was the age of the laser. I was working with the doctor preparing clients' skin for surgery and laser treatments, and taking care of them after their procedures. Some of the surgeries took months to heal, and I'd be changing bandages for weeks. I became extremely innovative, creating custom regimens for women whose skin couldn't handle everyday products, and I witnessed their skin transform. To this day, the healing power of skin astounds and inspires me. I'd watch women who'd undergone extreme face-lifts go from completely swollen and unrecognizable to absolutely healthy and healed. I built a successful business, with a busy schedule and a loyal clientele.

Before long, I met and fell in love with an incredible man, and we decided to move together to his hometown of Los Angeles. I sold my clinic to the doctor and got married. For a period of time after moving to L.A., I worked for a skin-care company in product development and was the director of education. I educated doctors and surgeons on the efficacy of the line and its ingredients, along with how it could support their business and treatments. My passion for product development began here. During this time, innovations in ingredients and technology were making products ever more effective. Vitamin C, retinoic acid, and alpha hydroxy acids could give clients the visible results they were looking for.

I enjoyed my work; however, the travel associated with it became overwhelming, so I again set up an esthetics office with a cosmetic surgeon in Santa Monica. At the time, he was the top surgeon in his field, and his clients included major celebrities. This doctor gave me the tools and inspiration I needed to fully pursue my dreams and career goals. He saw how I was constantly mixing and matching product lines to get my clients results. So one day he took me aside and said, "The only way you're going to make a difference is through innovation. You have six different skin-care lines here. Learn from them and make your own."

So I did. From that day on, I started to develop my own product collection. My first product was Quench Hydrating Serum, and to this day it's one of my top-three sellers. My clinic was very successful, but before I knew it—surprise!—I was pregnant. I worked really hard and knew that I couldn't keep the same hours with a baby. So I began seeing my clients at home, and all the while I continued to develop my product collection.

I had my little boy when I was 32 and spent a few years at home taking care of him. Then I decided that it was time for me to do my own thing: *totally* my own. My idea was to deliver the results you could get in a doctor's office but put my own stamp on it. I wanted to open a place where women and men would feel comfortable going: a place that would not only change their skin but also empower them to take control of their lives. I wanted to be able to develop partnerships with clients so that they could come in once a month or more frequently and achieve all of their skin-health goals.

In the spring of 2004, I opened my own full-service medi-skin clinic: Kate Somerville Skin Health Experts on Melrose Place in Los Angeles. There were just a few of us: two estheticians, Kyoko and Kimberly; my nurse, Sarah; my creative right hand, Tracy; and our Medical Director, Dr. Viguen Movsesian. Together we were able to build treatments and protocols for every age, ethnicity, and skin type. We gave hope to those who couldn't find solutions to their skin concerns anywhere else.

Not long after we opened, word spread throughout the entertainment industry that we could solve skin issues *and* be trusted. So within a year of opening, we had a list of celebrity clients who depended on us for healthy, radiant skin. What we were doing also caught the attention of the media. Television shows such as *Access Hollywood* and those on E!—along with *Allure, Vogue,* and *People* magazines—began reporting on our products and services. Stories about my strategies and skin philosophy soon appeared in other major media outlets, and before I knew it, I was the "guru of glow."

While my career was reaching new heights, my mother was swiftly declining. The tables had turned: she no longer consumed drugs and alcohol; they consumed her. My mom was homeless and living on the streets. Over time, her addictions stole her possessions, her spirit, and ultimately, her life. Thankfully, I got to see her and make peace with her before she passed away a few years ago. Today, she lives in my heart as I want to remember her: the loving mother who was an angel to so many but struggled in this world.

Because my personal life has often been so challenging, it's no surprise that I've always thrown myself into my work. It's been a place where I could go and *let go*—a place where I could create and have some control. After opening the clinic (which, by the way, doesn't look like a "clinic"—it's gorgeous and glamorous and comfortable and cozy all at once), I got serious about my product collection. I began to innovate and develop, with the help of my clients. Women and men of every skin type and concern came to see us every day, so they were the perfect group to tell me what I needed to create, and then to test it and tell me if it worked.

I'm not a chemist, but I knew exactly what I wanted and needed. So I immersed myself in the process, learned, and emerged with a product line that met my needs as a clinician and those of my clients. In the fall of 2006, we launched the Kate Somerville product collection . . . truly a dream come true for me! At first it was sold just at my clinic and a few boutiques and luxury spas, but now it's sold worldwide. I can hardly believe it; sometimes I have to pinch myself. To know that I'm helping people all over the world is one of the greatest pleasures I get from this job.

The truth is, many companies that create beauty products are really just marketing firms. They get formulas from a faraway lab and slap their labels on them. I truly believe this is what separates my brand, my products, and what my team and I do from all the rest of the stuff out there. My products don't get on the shelves unless they're needed by my clients and tested by real people at my clinic. We only create products that work and help, that my clients can trust, and that I believe in.

This book is no different; in fact, it's the latest extension of my skin-care mission. It's my way of being able to touch, help, and heal the skin of anyone who needs it. The act of helping women and men discover their best selves, starting with a focus on their skin, is truly the most inspiring work of my life. I enjoy educating and offering straightforward advice for real people with real concerns.

Whatever the obstacle, big or small, I want to give you the legs you need to jump beyond it, or the wings you need to fly over it. Within these pages, I'm giving you the knowledge and strategies I've learned and applied over the years. And the exciting thing for me is that I'm *still* learning!

My goal is to offer you nothing less than *Complexion Perfection!*—so turn the page to begin.

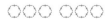

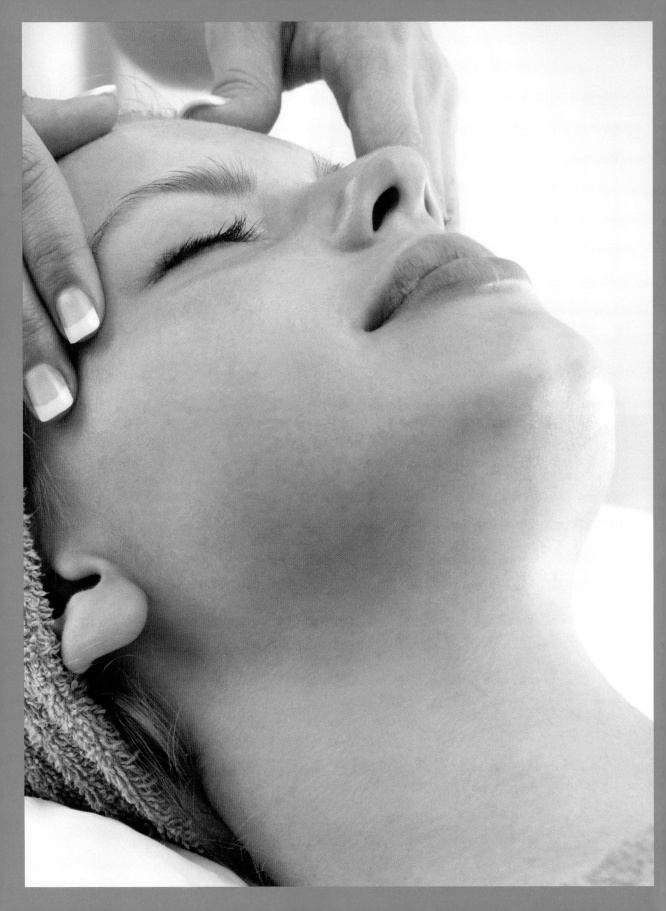

PART I

Complexion Direction!

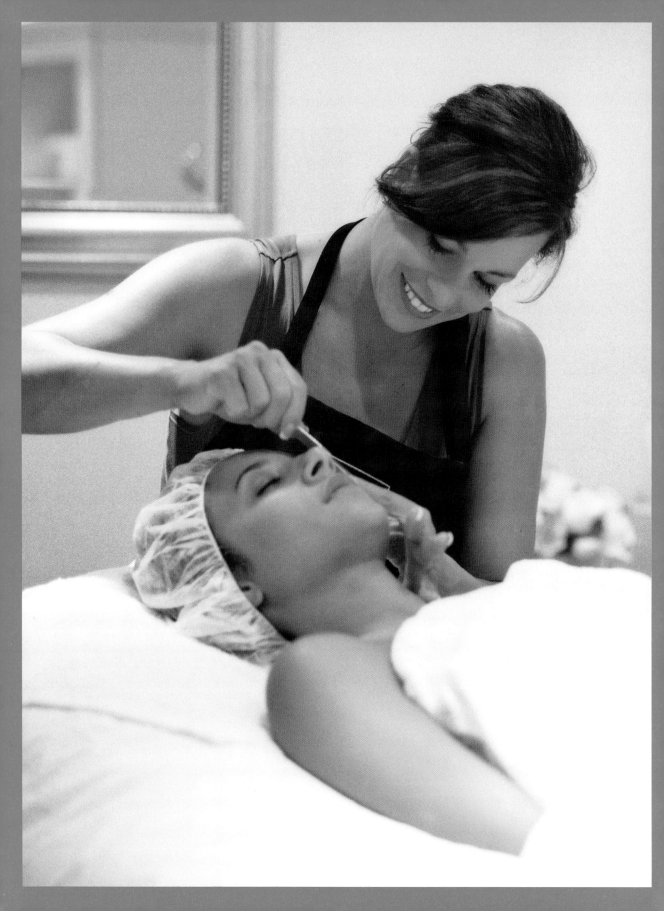

CHAPTER 1

Skin-ology 101

I've traveled the globe from New York to London to Los Angeles talking to men and women about their skin. Like these individuals, I'm sure you have a strong grasp of your own skin. You can tell me where you have lines, veins, spots, or clogged pores; whether you're sensitive or dry; or if you're hormonal and breaking out. But the truth is, there's so much more to your skin than meets your eye.

You may be familiar with some biology or buzzwords such as *collagen, elastin, free radicals, fine lines, light treatments,* and *laser peels.* But chances are, you don't *really* understand your skin, how it functions, and what lies beneath it. And if you're anything like me, you'll be tempted to skim this chapter or even skip ahead, but knowledge is power! So get out your yellow highlighter, ladies and gentlemen. Snuggle up with a good book (this one!), sip some green tea (it's good for your skin), and let's get gabbing. A better understanding of skin biology will help you understand just how all of the lotions, potions, and magic machines we'll talk about later can work for you.

Getting to Know Your Skin

Human skin is truly amazing. Despite my years in the business, I'm wowed by this majestic organ every day: what it does, how it heals, and just how beautiful it can be. If you think you're good at multitasking, trust me, you don't hold a candle to your skin. It serves hundreds of functions, including providing a supple, strong barrier between you and the outside world; receiving touch; and detoxifying your body.

Culturally, skin identifies our ethnic heritage, links us to our family, and is a blank canvas we sometimes color to express our individuality. Like it or not, our skin is a large part of what makes a first impression, and it's also what sets us apart as humans. Unlike our pooches, parakeets, or pet lizards, we're among the rare members of the animal kingdom whose skin is not protected by fur, feathers, or scales. We're born with skin that beams with light, what artist Vincent van Gogh characterized as "fresh from God." At birth, our physical shell seems too delicate to do everything we ask of it, but it's more than up to the job.

Here are some of the daily functions of our skin:

- Prevents our bodies from absorbing many toxins, including harmful chemicals and microorganisms in the environment

- Regulates our temperature by opening and closing blood vessels as needed, and by making perspiration that evaporates to cool us down

- Provides a waterproof shield so that our vital nutrients don't leak out of our body

- Gets rid of some of the body's waste products, including salt and ammonia, through sweat

- Helps protect us from sun damage by manufacturing melanin that tans it

- Produces oil to keep itself comfortable

- When exposed to sunlight, synthesizes the vitamin D we need for strong bones and healthy organs

- Houses our sense of touch, which allows us to enjoy a tickle or a hug and also alerts us of potential damage to our body via pain or discomfort

- Self-heals the cuts, nicks, scrapes, stings, punctures, bruises, burns, and blisters that we inflict on it day to day

Our skin can also reflect our state of health, since it's our body's biggest and fastest-growing organ. Get this: If you could unzip your skin, step out of it, and put it on a scale, it would weigh between six and nine pounds and cover an area of about 20 square feet (depending on your height and size). In other words, it would weigh about as much as a lapdog and could replace the carpet of a small yoga studio! It's also the largest organ that's visible to the outside world, so if you're not getting certain minerals in your diet or you're eating lots of junk, it will absolutely show up on your skin for you (and others) to see.

Think about it. How often do we say that people look pale or flushed, or that they have dark circles under their eyes? We know from those telltale signs that they might not be feeling their best or treating their body as well as they should. And how many times have we looked at our own faces in the mirror and thought, *I've **got** to get more sleep!* (I'm on the go so much, I've done this a lot.) But the opposite also shows—when we treat our body well, we see the rewards. We all know how we can glow after working out, when we're on vacation, or after a good night's rest.

Similarly, our emotions show up here, too. The blemish before a big date we're nervous about? The pink flush when we're embarrassed? That's skin responding to our stress levels. Then there are other, more serious dermatological conditions, such as eczema, that studies have shown are linked to chronic stress or traumatic events. Research has actually found that stress can make skin more prone to allergies. One reason is that stress can suppress our immune function, leaving us more vulnerable. We'll talk more about this later.

The truth is that our skin impacts how we feel about ourselves and how others view us. I've seen it over and over again: a glowing, healthy complexion leaves us feeling attractive and ready for anything, while an imperfect or ailing one can make us not want to face the world. And in case you think that you're alone in this, I can tell you from experience that some of the most recognized faces in the world—those celebrities you see at movie premieres and on the pages of magazines—have exactly the same concerns. Many of them are my clients, and I know how they feel and what they go through.

Our skin is also a dramatic indicator of time's passage. Subtle changes over the decades take us from the gorgeous dewy skin of infancy; through the frustrations of adolescent acne, the hormonal pigment problems of pregnancy, and the fine wrinkles of midlife; and then into the deeply etched face of our golden years.

It may come as a shock to you to learn that our bodies technically start "aging" when we're in our early 20s as cell production begins to slow down. Of course we're all going to age, but how and when our skin shows the signs of aging are subject to a number of factors, most of which we can actually influence and increasingly have control over. For example:

— *Genetics* are responsible for more than just your blue eyes and freckles or your olive complexion. The DNA that's passed on to you also contributes to whether or not you have oily skin or are prone to breakouts, and it sets your biological timeline. Look at your parents and grandparents for some clues as to how your skin is going to age. The good news is that you are not destined to live with these imperfections—there are now treatments and products available to influence their development and to minimize them if you so desire. So while "kin skin" is inherited, you can still work to change what you've got.

— *Hormones* have a major impact on the skin at just about every stage of life. When they start surging in adolescence, they can cause acne. Later, some birth control pills can cause breakouts in women, while others can help clear up acne. Pregnancies can result in hormone-related hyperpigmentation; you've heard it called the "pregnancy mask." Then as menopause sets in, estrogen levels dip and skin becomes significantly drier, more fragile, and loses elasticity. And, in a cruel twist of fate, it can get acne again!

When we speak of hormones, we do tend to think of the sex hormones such as estrogen and testosterone, but there are others such as cortisol—a stress hormone—that also impact our skin. But have no fear: I'm going to tell you how we can deal with all of this hormone-related complexion chaos.

— *Free radicals.* Like the radical revolutionaries you've watched on the History Channel, these radicals also wreak havoc, only they do it to your body. They're a natural part of your bodily function, but they do speed up aging. They are a certain type of oxygen molecule that causes a chain reaction of damage—oxidation—to your cells. It's not just human cells that are affected by oxidation; in fact, you can see this process in action in your kitchen. Notice how when you first buy a piece of fresh meat, it's bright red in color. But if you let it sit in your fridge for a few days, oxidation turns it brown or gray. And the brown patch after you've bitten an apple? Also the work of free radicals.

The antidote to oxidation is the appropriately named "antioxidant"—a wide variety of vitamins and minerals found in fresh foods and nutritional supplements. Over the years I've learned so much about the connection of a healthy diet to glowing skin. Well, the reverse is true in that an unhealthy diet deficient in antioxidants is going to contribute to the aging caused by free radicals. We can also fight free radicals and promote cell recovery with topical applications of antioxidants.

— *Lifestyle.* For most of us, free-radical damage is caused by pollutants, too much sun, and other environmental challenges, such as overexposure to wind or intense heat and cold. Unhealthy habits (like drinking too much alcohol, getting too little sleep, smoking, and living with chronic stress) also take their toll on your skin.

Science has recently proven how a healthy lifestyle dramatically impacts how well we age. While we may be getting older in years, we can actually look and feel better. We frequently hear "40 is the new 30," or even "60 is the new 40." One thing I do believe, as Gertrude Stein is rumored to have said, "We are always the same age inside."

You might have heard of or even taken the RealAge Test that author and television personality Dr. Mehmet Oz is fond of talking about. This quiz says that there really can be a difference between how many birthdays you've had and your *real* age. Still, no matter how fit you are, your skin can betray your years if you don't take all the right steps to keep it equally healthy.

The Anatomy of Your Skin

Now let's break down the anatomy of your skin, one layer at a time.

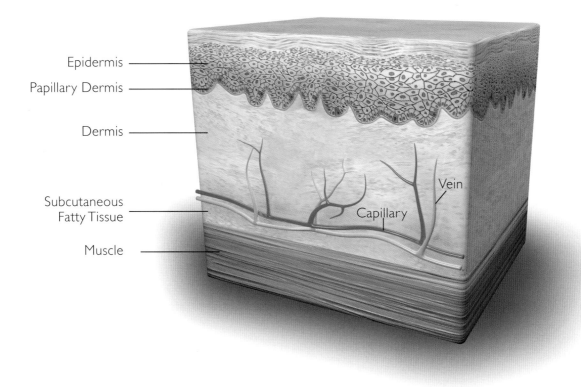

Epidermis

Papillary Dermis

Dermis

Subcutaneous Fatty Tissue

Muscle

Vein

Capillary

I. THE EPIDERMIS

The epidermis is the top layer; it's what you see. It's thinnest around your eyes and thickest on the soles of your feet. It doesn't have any blood vessels and is fed oxygen and nutrients from the deeper layers. However, it does contain cells that form your skin's immune system. That's a good thing, since a 2007 study funded by the National Institutes of Health discovered hundreds of species of bacteria on human skin, and 8 percent of them were unknown to scientists! Think of your epidermal cells as skin soldiers, since they're your first line of defense against enemies.

The epidermis has five layers of cells and millions of skin cells per square inch. Every day, new cells are born. The cells are shaped like little columns and are made in the lowest layer, and then they divide and push up into the higher layers. As the cells move upward, they flatten out and eventually die. The top cell dictates what the one being born beneath it is going to be like and what it does. So for healthy skin, you need to not only get rid of the damaged cells on top but also manage what's going on below.

This whole process of new cells working their way from the bottom to the top takes about 30 days, although it slows down considerably as you age. The dead cells spend another two weeks on the surface of your skin before naturally sloughing off as a new layer of cells is pushed to the top. The surface of your skin—the skin the world sees—is actually made up of dead, flat cells. Yuck! As you might imagine, those dead cells are largely responsible for your skin looking dull and lifeless. They also build up around your pores and wrinkles, making them look larger. Getting rid of the dead layer when it's ready and turning over those skin cells are crucial for a brighter complexion. Journalists constantly ask me about the most important step in skin care. There is no one thing, as everything works together. But I do believe that exfoliation is key because you see immediate results from it.

The bottom layer of your epidermis makes melanin, the pigment that gives your skin its color. It's also what goes into overdrive when you're working on your tan. During exposure to ultraviolet rays, melanin activates, producing a tan in an attempt to protect your skin from damage by those rays. As the decades roll by, the cells that make melanin die off, and your skin becomes more susceptible to burning. This puts you at an increased risk for signs of aging and skin cancer.

2. THE DERMIS

Now, beneath the epidermis is the dermis. It's much thicker than the epidermis and is rich with blood vessels and nerves. The dermis also sends nutrients and moisture up to the epidermis to keep it healthy. Just like the epidermis, the dermis is thinnest around your eyes and thickest on your feet.

In recent decades, we experts have learned so much about the importance of this layer, especially with regard to aging. So what exactly is going on here? This dermal layer has a lot of responsibilities. It's made up of connective tissues which are composed of proteins you've probably heard of: collagen and elastin. The collagen gives the skin its fullness and form, while the elastin gives skin its snap—a rubber-band-like resilience. Cells called fibroblasts make collagen and elastin on a continual basis. They're all bathed in hyaluronic acid, a cellular lipid and lubricant that holds water, giving your skin texture, bounce, and a youthful look.

The dermis also houses your hair follicles and oil glands, although there are none of these on the palms of your hands, the soles of your feet, or your lips—and that's one of the reasons why these areas can be so dry. A superhighway of nerves responsible for your sense of touch, pain, itch, and temperature is also situated here. Hair, sweat, and oil all reach the surface of the skin via pores, which begin in this layer. While pores have a job to do, most of my clients have a love/hate relationship with them.

So, when you're "Sweatin' to the Oldies," chatting with a crush and start to blush, feeling goose bumps after a case of déjà vu, or suffering a pre-wedding acne attack, it *all* starts in the dermis. And guess what? The signs of aging start here, too. Here's why: When you're young, your dermis can stretch and then bounce back into shape. But as you age, the collagen and elastin break down faster than your fibroblasts (the cells that make them) can produce these proteins. The number of fibroblasts you have also shrinks, so the whole network becomes more brittle and no longer snaps back like it used to. And that, combined with gravity, causes wrinkles to form.

Hyaluronic acid also decreases over time, as do the number of oil and sweat glands, which contributes to dry skin and aging. But wait—don't let this get you down. We live in such an exciting time and can do something about all of this. There are products and treatments available that can penetrate this layer to build collagen and repair elasticity and replace hyaluronic acid. Woo-hoo! These are the things that keep me (and my actor clients) in business!

3. SUBCUTANEOUS TISSUE

Although technically not skin, the layer of fat and connective tissue that lies between your skin and muscles does have an effect on your complexion and how it looks. This tissue supplies energy and is a protective cushion and insulator for your body. It has larger blood vessels and nerves and is important, as it regulates the temperature of your skin and of your entire body.

Subcutaneous fat covers our muscles and bones and is loosely attached to them. The thickness of this layer varies throughout the body and from person to person. On the face, this layer tends to get thinner in most of us as we age, so our skin looks less plump and smooth, and underlying structures and veins show through more. Unfortunately, this is not true on other parts of our body, and we can all blame this subcutaneous fat for cellulite. Mary, my bodyworker, has magic hands and helps me work on that. (Massage helps, but I'm still hoping for a miracle in the cellulite department!)

Turning that "frown upside down" is the job of our facial muscles. There are several muscle groups under the skin and subcutaneous tissue that stretch in layers over our facial bones. When we smile, frown, wink, whistle, or pout, we're using these muscle groups. We also use them to chew and swallow. Over time, these repetitive motions and expressions contribute to forming the familiar lines we see on our faces.

As we age, we also lose facial muscle mass and tone. Gravity gets into the act and those loose muscles start to head south, taking our skin with them. At one time, surgical face-lifts were the only real answer to this problem. But now we have treatments that actually function as a gym for the face, lifting and firming the actual muscles.

Skin to the Future

The treatments we have available today are just the beginning compared to what's coming. The Human Genome Project that was published in 2003 has opened up a world of possibilities for our health and our health care. Doctors can already tell from looking at our genes if we're at risk for certain diseases and head some of them off with preventive medicine. This also offers amazing potential for the way we treat skin. I can foresee a time when, in the not-too-distant future, you'll walk into a clinic like mine and have a swab of DNA taken. After it's been analyzed, we'll be able to plan a skin-care regimen to deal with the aging issues you've inherited, address what deficiencies you have, and know if you're genetically prone to skin cancers or other serious conditions. This will be the age of truly personalized skin care. Pure gene-ius!

In the meantime, here's something hot off the scientific presses: Researchers at Stanford University School of Medicine have discovered that blocking just one protein can reverse aging in skin. So far they have only experimented on mice, but the results were startling. In only two weeks, the scientists reversed aging skin to youthful skin. Can you imagine the future implications for humans?

While we're on the topic of exciting scientific breakthroughs, let's talk about stem cells. Researchers have found that babies in the womb can heal from injuries and surgeries without scarring because their stem cells cause regeneration at an incredibly fast rate. A peptide that affects stem cells has been derived from a substance found in umbilical cords, which has exciting possibilities for anti-aging skin care. One day we really may be able to have a face as soft and smooth as a baby's bottom! And I believe that's just around the corner. This is why I say we live in such an exciting time regarding skin care.

So as you try to navigate through the overwhelming world of today's (and tomorrow's) skin care, with its limitless lists of ingredients, treatments, products, peels, lasers, and lights, I'd like to simplify things for you by arming you with my instruction manual. The next chapter covers the five most important elements for healthy skin at every age. So flip the page for your forever "guide to the glow."

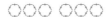

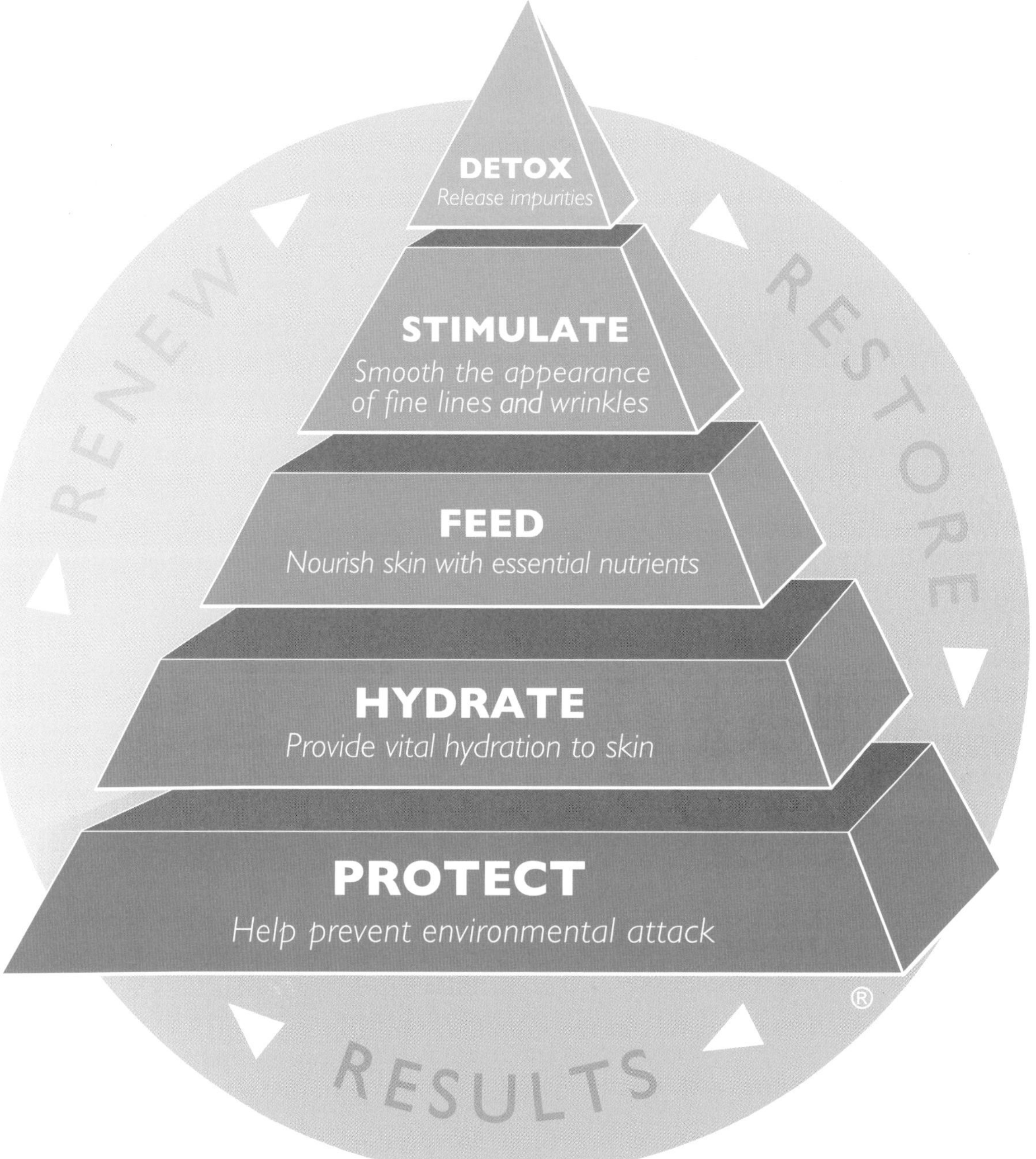
DETOX
Release impurities
STIMULATE
Smooth the appearance of fine lines and wrinkles
FEED
Nourish skin with essential nutrients
HYDRATE
Provide vital hydration to skin
PROTECT
Help prevent environmental attack
RENEW
RESTORE
RESULTS
®

CHAPTER 2

My Skin Health Pyramid®— Five Principles

What changes skin? How do we achieve healthy skin? Well, here's an analogy. My husband, Landa, is a talented musician. Apart from creativity, like all musicians he knows there are basic formulas that make up a catchy chorus; a great melody; and, ultimately, a good song you can sing along to. Healthy, radiant skin is no different. So what's the universal formula for this? How do you get it and then keep it? How do you get skin that you want to sing along to?

I first started thinking about this a few years ago, when I was with a friend at a cabin in Big Bear. It was a lazy day, and we were bundled up, sipping tea, watching the snow flurries outside the window, and brainstorming what would become this book. At this point, I'd been working on skin for almost 15 years, and time and time again I'd seen my clients' skin transform. My friend swore to me that until we met, she'd tried everything—but it wasn't until she did what I told her that her skin transformed from acne prone and sensitive to healthy and vibrant. As we talked about what worked for her and what didn't, this casual discussion turned into a dedicated research session. Then my mission became to put down on paper what had worked for me for years.

I began asking myself, *What is the formula for healthy skin?* I focused on the big picture: *What do I do to change skin? What's required for skin to be as healthy as possible at any age? And if it's not healthy and radiant, what do I do to get those results?*

I truly believe that your skin can look and act healthy at any age, provided that it's cared for on every level. I reviewed hundreds of client cases in my head and hundreds more when I got back to my office. I looked at charts, "before" and "after" photos, treatment programs, and suggested regimens. I began to recognize a clear pattern: Regardless of skin's condition, age, ethnicity, or concern, there was a method behind my success in treating it. And there was a formula for achieving and maintaining complexion perfection. I immediately put pen to paper and outlined the strategy I'd applied to my clients over the years. I organized these principles into the Kate Somerville Skin Health Pyramid®, and conceptually modeled it after the U.S. Department of Agriculture's Food Guide Pyramid because it was so simple and easy to understand.

The Skin Health Pyramid is organized into five basic principles: **Protect, Hydrate, Feed, Stimulate,** and **Detox.** When all principles are applied, the result is a healthy, clear, radiant complexion. That's why when I meet a new client, I examine her skin and break down her current regimen, and then I ask myself, *What part of the pyramid is this person missing?* When reading about the pyramid in the following pages, ask yourself the same question. What parts of the pyramid are you leaving out? What elements are you following? I do this myself. When my own skin is a mess, I can usually get to the bottom of things fairly quickly by taking inventory of my personal application of the pyramid.

Each element of the Skin Health Pyramid has two different dimensions—external and internal—that fit in the big picture to foster healthy skin and then a healthy *you*. (As you're reading along, please note that I mention some ingredients and treatments that I'll explain more fully in the following chapters.)

Level 1: Protect

Protection is the first level of my Skin Health Pyramid because it keeps your skin healthy, and healthy skin is the foundation of beautiful skin. If you don't protect your skin, then the issues you fix will come right back again. Protecting your skin from every angle is the unequivocal foundation of my philosophy.

EXTERNAL

External protection is the most important element for healthy skin. We've all been coached to look under our arms, on our bums, or anywhere with limited exposure to the sun and other environmental factors—and we find that the skin there tends to be smooth and soft, with fewer lines, wrinkles, spots, or other unsavory stamps of damage.

The sun is a marvelous thing; we need it, as well as the vitamin D it stimulates in our body, in order to function. For me, there is nothing more enjoyable than walking barefoot on the warm sand next to the ocean. Unfortunately, the sun degrades our collagen and elastin and affects our body's ability to create healthy new cells. What we generally associate with skin aging is less a matter of chronology and more a free-radical issue. The free radicals produced by UV (ultraviolet) rays become highly reactive and ultimately cause damage to our DNA strands, causing the genetic structure of our cells to change. Those cells are no longer perfect copies of the ones that came before; the new, imperfect cells then begin to influence each consecutive new cell in the form of an unhealthy structure.

UV exposure can also cause photoaging and skin cancers. Here's how it works. The sun emits three wavelengths of ultraviolet radiation: UVA, UVB, and UVC. Most UVC rays are absorbed by the ozone layer, so they're no threat to us. The other two are another story. UVA rays, which are consistently strong all the time, account for about 95 percent of the sun's rays that reach Earth. They cause overactive melanin cells and the breakdown of collagen and elastin. UVBs vary in strength depending on the time of day and time of year and are what cause sunburns. The bottom line is that sunburn is an unmistakable indication that you've experienced severe damage. Ouch!

As for cancer, both UVA and UVB rays can be responsible for it, but UVAs may be the more dangerous of the two. Although they don't burn you like UVBs do, they intensify the cancer-causing effects of UVBs, penetrate deeper, and more severely affect skin cells.

Many clients walk in my door and ask me to take away or reverse something they don't like about their skin, and usually what they don't like could have been avoided by staying out of the sun! Those few minutes in the sun here and there add up to a lifetime of damage to the skin.

Some of us have more melanin in our skin and can handle more sun exposure, but that doesn't mean we can avoid wearing sunscreen. For example, my mom was part Native American, and I inherited her olive complexion and penchant for sun worshipping. In my 20s, I loved to bask in the rays at the beach. I thought, *I'm olive; I can handle this.* But my skin couldn't—in my early 30s, I started to notice lines around my eyes and on my forehead. Yet where I really noticed the sun damage was on my chest. So a word of advice: wear sunscreen on your treasure chest! There are fewer skin cells per inch on your neck and chest, so they tend to be thinner and more prone to aging and damage. Just like your face, they must be protected. Now I never leave the house without applying sunscreen with at least an SPF (sun protection factor) of 30, and I strongly suggest you do the same—even in winter and on cloudy days.

Sunscreen today is better than ever, as there have been innovations in technology that effectively protect and nourish the skin. I recommend looking for sunscreens with ingredients that contain either physical or chemical blocks, and always look for broad-spectrum protection, which means protection from all UV rays.

One of my favorite forms of sun protection is mineral makeup. (I use the Jane Iredale brand; Jane pioneered the concept, but there are many other good ones out there, including Bare Escentuals.) The minerals that comprise these powders protect against UV rays—they create a physical barrier between your skin and the sun and usually have an SPF of 15 to 22. These products are a great alternative for those with really sensitive skin and the acne prone. If you don't like to apply powder directly to your skin, add a few sprinkles into your liquid sunscreen. This will give you added protection, along with very natural coverage.

Apart from sunscreen and mineral makeup, there are topical ingredients that help protect the skin from the sun and other environmental factors, such as pollution. Make sure that moisturizers and serums contain free-radical-fighting antioxidants, including vitamins C and E and green-tea extract.

You also need to cover up. Now, I don't believe in living like a mummy—after all, my parents were hippies! I just recommend making smart choices. Wear a hat when you're out in the sun for any length of time and especially in the middle of the day. A hat with a two- or three-inch brim all around will protect your face, neck, and ears. (Note that a visor or baseball cap will shade your face but leave your ears and the back of your neck vulnerable.) Tightly woven fabric such as canvas offers better protection than mesh fabric or straw. Wraparound sunglasses protect not only your eyes, but also the delicate skin around them. And the less you squint in the sun, the less you'll contribute to wrinkles forming.

Perhaps the smart rule to live by is the Cancer Council Australia slogan: "Slip on a shirt, slop on some sunscreen, and slap on a hat."

INTERNAL

While there isn't a sunscreen supplement (yet!), there are certain foods and ingredients that increase the natural SPF of your skin. There's a reason watermelon is so popular in the summer months: nature intended it that way. Eating watermelon can actually boost your SPF by several factors. Pomegranate, which has been used as a multidimensional medicinal fruit for years, is also proven to boost your natural protection factor. Foods or supplements that contain essential fatty acids, such as omega-3, strengthen the skin's natural barrier function and also help protect the skin from within.

Level 2: Hydrate

Hydration follows protection in the pyramid, and I love to talk about this topic. Sadly, despite its crucial importance, I find that so many of my clients are missing this step. Seriously! They know to moisturize their skin and to drink water, both of which are important—but they aren't *hydrating* their skin, which is something totally different.

Hydration means getting water into the skin cells; moisturizing means locking it there by applying a cream or lotion on top of the hydrated skin. Think about your skin as a piece of dry leather (and leather is, after all, animal skin). If you put a drop of water on it, the wet patch will plump up but will soon dry out again if left alone. If you apply an oily preservative over the wet patch, however, it will remain plump. Both hydration and moisturization are truly necessary because more-hydrated cells are healthier cells; they look and function better.

Our cells need water to function efficiently; without the proper hydration, they die. Think of how supple and firm a grape is. Now think of a wrinkly, hard raisin. The difference between the two is simple: the raisin is dried out and no longer holds water. We are born plump, juicy grapes and have to work hard not to become raisins.

We need to do several things in order to keep skin as hydrated as possible. The products we choose should contain ingredients that act as:

- **Humectants,** to attract water to the skin cell
- **Occlusives,** that keep hydration from evaporating
- **Emollients,** that add lubrication to the epidermis

Those of us with dry skin will need more humectants, and those of us who are acne prone will require fewer emollients. This is one reason why one person might think that a particular moisturizer is the best out there, yet it may clog someone else's pores. We'll talk more about specific hydrating ingredients in a later chapter.

I'm a huge believer in hyaluronic acid as a topical ingredient because it functions to hold water in, and I'm so glad that it's becoming more widely available in skin-care products. Hyaluronic acid is a powerful humectant, occlusive, and emollient. It's unique in that it binds water into the skin cells and helps them hold a thousand times their weight in water. When we're children, we heal faster, and one of the reasons for this is that our cells hold a higher percentage of water and hyaluronic acid. Stores of hyaluronic acid slowly deplete as we age, and our bodies' production of it declines. This is why it's crucial that we supplement with it topically and internally.

External hydration is not only about what you're doing to bring in and lock in moisture, but also about what you're doing to keep from dehydrating. Dehydration greatly affects the barrier function. If you overexfoliate with ingredients that are too harsh or overtreat your skin, you can compromise its external barrier and leave it unprotected. Water will then evaporate very quickly, leaving your skin dry, dehydrated, and prone to sensitivity and infection.

It's not always easy to deliver hydration deep into the skin cells, since the epidermis doesn't have the power to pull it down as completely as necessary. So external hydration must be complemented with internal hydration.

Most of us know that we need to drink water to stay hydrated: the rule of thumb (although studies are inconclusive) is generally eight glasses a day, and more if we are highly physically active, work outdoors, or live in a very hot climate. But recently I've been asking myself, *What **is** healthy hydration?* There seems to be so much controversy about water sources, bottling, levels of purity, distilled versus not, and so forth. My stance is that we should do research and make the decision that is best for us. Even if purified by a filter, I believe that we have little control over what gets into the water during the transportation process. Certain metals and impurities can be filtered out, but what about chemicals, drugs, and other toxic materials that aren't caught by the filter?

I encourage you to look into your local water supply and get to know what's in it. Your local Department of Water should provide you with specific data on what chemicals and impurities are in your water supply. You may then decide whether you want to use a home filtration system or would rather get bottled water from a company that you believe has the highest-quality product. (When my father-in-law was going through an intense, Eastern-medicine program to fight prostate cancer, for instance, he only drank Penta water. This brand is ultrapurified, and the company claims that it helps fight free radicals.)

Along with drinking enough water, supplementing with fish oil and flaxseed oil for essential omega-3 fatty acids works to hydrate and lock moisture into skin cells. Hyaluronic-acid supplements, when combined with coenzyme Q_{10}, are also incredibly effective in attracting more water to the skin cells and then locking it in by preventing evaporation.

Healthy internal hydration is also about making sure that you don't dehydrate yourself and your cells. Diuretics can help reduce excess water retention and puffiness, but don't go overboard with them. Coffee, black tea, and sodas can dehydrate, as caffeine pulls the moisture content out of skin cells—and, you'll notice, makes you visit the bathroom more frequently. Carbonated drinks, in a roundabout way, trick your body into thinking that it has more water, so you tend to hydrate less. Alcohol is extremely dehydrating as well.

Simple sugars such as high-fructose corn syrup and refined white sugar take a lot of water to metabolize. High-protein and high-fiber foods, although essential for your health, also require a lot of it to process. This is all the more reason to drink plenty of water. I personally carry around a big bottle of it with me everywhere, every day.

Skin-ny Dipping

I first discovered the fantastic healing benefits of baths when I was struggling with an awful flare-up of eczema all over and just couldn't seem to shake it. I met a dream dermatologist who told me to put my prescription creams away and get in the tub. He said, "We have to put you back into the womb." Considering all of the struggles I'd had with my mom, if he only knew how true that was!

He had me bathe every morning and every night for 20 minutes. My mind moves a million miles an hour, and at first each minute *felt* like an hour. But I began to consider my bath time as an opportunity to slow my mind down and care for myself. The doctor also had me slather lotion all over myself as soon as I got out of the tub. To this day, whenever I have a flare-up, this routine helps get my eczema under control—and anyone who suffers from dry, itchy, or irritated skin may find it useful as well. (**Note:** I think it's best not to add anything to the bath unless it's fragrance-free oil, a milk product, oatmeal, or Epsom salts.)

Level 3: Feed

Our bodies are miracle machines. But in order for them to function properly, they need proper nutrition that provides the most efficient fuel. We need to feed our skin from the inside out *and* the outside in.

EXTERNAL

While our skin may be our largest organ, it's the least vital one. Our bodies are designed to deliver energy and nutrients in a hierarchy, providing essential nutrients to the most vital organs such as the heart, liver, kidneys, and brain first, leaving—you guessed it—the skin in last place. It gets whatever's left over, if anything. And these days, because of the declining nutritional content of our food supply, there usually isn't much left over. However, our bodies are brilliant. Our skin is literally a sponge and can absorb up to 60 percent of certain nutrients that we deliver externally.

So my advice is: feed your face!

Topical vitamins, minerals, antioxidants, and essential oils have been found to be incredibly efficient in feeding the skin. Vitamins C and E are proven antioxidants, which fight those free radicals that cause damage to healthy cells and DNA. Topical vitamin A, in the form of retinoic acid or retinol, helps break up skin cells that are irregularly stacked—this encourages cells to turn over and creates smoother skin with fewer lines. Minerals can also be a great help: copper can aid in strengthening and supporting the structural matrix of the skin, stimulating the production of collagen and elastin; while zinc, used topically, is an anti-inflammatory. Certain essential oils such as tea tree are known to help minimize oil production, which is incredibly useful for those who tend to have congested pores and blackheads due to excessively oily skin.

INTERNAL

What we put into our body is every bit as important as what we put onto our face. Most of us have known for years that what we eat ultimately affects every system in our bodies: our vision, our brain function, our immunity, our mood, our weight, our circulation, and our skin. Yet I don't think I really knew what eating healthfully was and to what extent it could impact the skin until my father-in-law adopted a particularly nutritious diet in order to fight cancer. (I'll tell you more of his incredible story later.) I couldn't believe the changes I saw in his skin. Spots disappeared, his redness turned into an inner radiance, and he looked ten years younger!

Since then, I've made changes in my own diet and have become committed to the idea of promoting good nutrition as an integral part of skin health. Clients who come in for a consultation are now given recommended dietary suggestions and modifications based on the condition of their skin. And many have made the same shift I have. That's why I've devoted an entire chapter of this book to food and eating, which I've titled "Beauty and the Buffet."

Level 4: Stimulate

The importance of stimulation becomes more and more evident as we gain knowledge about our skin's health and structure. And the stimulation of circulation—along with collagen and elastin and other processes that support a healthy cellular structure—becomes increasingly critical as we age.

EXTERNAL

I believe that one of the most effective ways to stimulate your skin externally is through topical ingredients such as vitamin A and peptides. Studies have shown that these ingredients stimulate fibroblasts; have the effect of reducing lines, smoothing texture, and minimizing pores and redness over time; strengthen elasticity; and add plumpness to the skin.

We know that sun damage affects the genetic structure of skin, causing cells to reproduce in unhealthy ways as the years go by. So not only do we need products that stimulate cells, we also need a delivery system that will carry the ingredients down to the levels where cells are formed. There have been tremendous advances in science and technology in this area for both products and treatments—for example, lasers and light treatments are wonderful for stimulating cellular renewal.

INTERNAL

Are there foods that stimulate collagen? You'd better believe it. As important as vitamin C is topically, it's just as essential internally for collagen synthesis. Trace minerals such as zinc and magnesium are key factors in the chemical processes that strengthen our tissue—pumpkin seeds are high in zinc and almonds are high in magnesium. And any foods that contain or promote omega-3 fatty acids, such as oily fish, walnuts, or flaxseeds will help support production of collagen.

Level 5: Detox

Just as our homes need care and cleaning, so do our bodies. They need a little upkeep each day, and every once in a while we need to really get in there and clean things out. Stuff accumulates over the days, weeks, and years. Eating, sleeping, stress—just living—can all create buildup that interferes with how our bodies look and function.

I've chosen my life, and it's not a slow-moving one. For the past few years I've been in a constant state of *go-go-go!* When I'm in tune with my pyramid, I schedule time to stop and to detox. But when I haven't done this, something inevitably stops me in my tracks. For example, a few years ago I was sidelined by mononucleosis. I could hardly get out of bed in the morning, and I believe it was because I wasn't supposed to. I'd been moving so fast for so long that this virus forced me to put on the brakes. So after months of feeling ill, I made a game plan: I would detoxify through exercise, nutrition, steaming, and massage.

When you detoxify, your body rids itself of toxins and impurities, oftentimes through the skin. Getting rid of this junk can give you more energy than you've ever had before, and it can leave your skin looking luminous. I have to give you one word of caution. Before you get to that luminous point, you may first break out in pimples or rashes as toxins release through the skin.

EXTERNAL

Externally detoxifying means a few things. One is cleansing daily—morning and night—with a cleanser that's right for your skin type. Those of you with dry, sensitive, or aging skin will want a gentle, sulfate-free cleanser; while those of you with acne need a cleanser with mild acids that gently exfoliate and help control oil production.

Exfoliating is another form of detoxifying. I suggest using an exfoliant on your face two or three times a week. Ridding your body of dead skin cells leaves the healthy cells on the surface and helps keep pores free of impurities. (My favorite exfoliant is ExfoliKate, a product in my line that uses natural fruit enzymes, gentle acids, and microbeads to do the job.)

A third way to detoxify is with facials: I recommend having them monthly, whether at a skin-care salon or doing them at home. They can rid your skin of impurities, dirt, debris, and bacteria that can be trapped in pores and create infection and breakouts.

For the body, dry brushing with a soft natural-fiber brush or loofah has been practiced for centuries—it's a great way to sweep away dead cells and tiny bumps and encourage the lymphatic system (a network of vessels, ducts, and organs) to release toxins. Do this before your shower or bath in the morning.

Skin-telligence:

DO YOU HAVE "CELL-PHONE FACE?" If you have breakouts or blemishes on the right side of your face—especially near your mouth and around the middle of the cheek—and you're right-handed, you most likely have "cell-phone face." Why? Well, your phone is seriously dirty. Think about how many times you pick it up after you've touched something, *anything* . . . and then it's stored in warm pockets, purses, and the like, which are perfect breeding grounds for gunk. All that bacteria gets smooshed into your pores as you jibber-jabber away. If you really want to be grossed out, studies have shown that your cell phone is dirtier than any other household object, including your toilet seat! So apart from causing pimples, your phone can carry germs that can actually make you sick. My advice is to carry antibacterial wipes with you and give your phone a thorough detox at least once a day.

Finally, sweat it out. As a society, we don't sweat nearly as much as we're designed to. In fact, we go out of our way *not* to sweat by living in air-conditioning, wearing antiperspirants, and not exerting ourselves. But it's so important to sweat because it is a way for toxins to get out of the body and is valuable for keeping pores clean. So work out until you can see the beads of sweat, sit in a sauna or steam room, or soak in a hot tub (your face will sweat) whenever you have the opportunity.

INTERNAL

There are a few simple things you can do on a daily basis to cleanse internally through certain drinks and foods: Pure, unfiltered cranberry juice diluted with water is a great way to cleanse your kidneys. A squeeze of lemon juice added to a glass of water and drunk a few times throughout the day will help neutralize excess acidity. And green tea is excellent for cleansing and immunity.

There are several methods to detoxify the body, and you should always consult a doctor or nutritionist before starting. Once or twice a year, I spend a week on a juice cleanse, but you don't necessarily have to do anything that severe. You can get a really effective cleanse by cutting out caffeine, alcohol, sugar, added salt, meat, and processed food from your diet for just three days. Drink only water, juice, or herbal tea; and load up on a variety of raw, fresh produce. (If you'd like to add in some protein, have a handful of nuts or some low-fat yogurt or cottage cheese.) The fiber in the fruits and vegetables acts like a brush throughout your intestinal system, sweeping away all the junk as it goes through. This kind of detox will not only cleanse your body, but it will

Skin-telligence:

PILLOW FRIGHT! If you could see the invisible zoo of microscopic bugs and dust mites that resides in your pillows and on their cases—in addition to the general buildup of bacteria, dirt, and debris—you'd change them every day. These little guys can cause a lot of skin problems, and those of you with sensitive-skin issues such as rosacea, acne, or eczema should pay special attention. There are some studies that actually link rosacea and some skin allergies to these little bugs. Which brings me to another point: if you know that your skin is sensitive, be aware of the detergent you use. You might want to switch to a product that's free of colors, chemicals, and fragrances, since all of these additives can add up to big problems.

also recalibrate your taste buds. They get used to whatever you feed them, and you can lose your taste for sugar and salt in as little as three days.

This next way of detoxing will only apply to some of you, but it's very important. *Stop smoking!* It's killing your skin. In fact, smoking is perhaps the single most detrimental thing you can do for your skin, even more than suntanning. Did you know that *smoker's face* is an actual term in the medical dictionary? That's because doctors can tell just by looking at the wrinkles, sallowness, constricted blood vessels, and premature aging that you're a smoker.

When you puff on a cigarette, you're drawing in more than 4,000 toxins, including carbon monoxide, ammonia, cyanide, butane, carbolic acid, arsenic, and cadmium. They make their way directly to your skin, clamping off capillaries, reducing oxygen supply, and ultimately slowing down collagen production. Smoking also eats up free-radical-fighting vitamin C in your body. A study of identical twins showed that the skin of the twin who smoked was between 25 and 40 percent thinner than the one who didn't. If that's not convincing enough, keep in mind that smoking causes wrinkling around your lips and around your eyes from squinting against the smoke.

The Skin Health Halo

Around the Skin Health Pyramid is something I call the "Skin Health Halo," because there is a component to healthy skin that's less obvious than enlarged pores or wrinkles. I've placed the pyramid inside this golden halo because when you apply all of the elements of the pyramid, it's essential to practice them with thoughtfulness. You can wear sunscreen, get facials, exercise, and eat healthfully; but if your spirit and mind aren't protected, hydrated, fed, stimulated, and detoxified, sooner or later your skin will reflect that. Your spiritual state, which can represent your state of satisfaction and happiness, must be all of these things for the greatest changes in the skin to happen, and for a truly radiant complexion to manifest.

Other, less tangible things can dramatically affect our skin: our mind and our emotions. In my experience, the mind has a powerful effect on our skin. Our emotional state impacts our skin tremendously, and is a part of the Skin Health Halo, so let's discuss just how we can change our skin by getting our emotions on track.

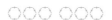

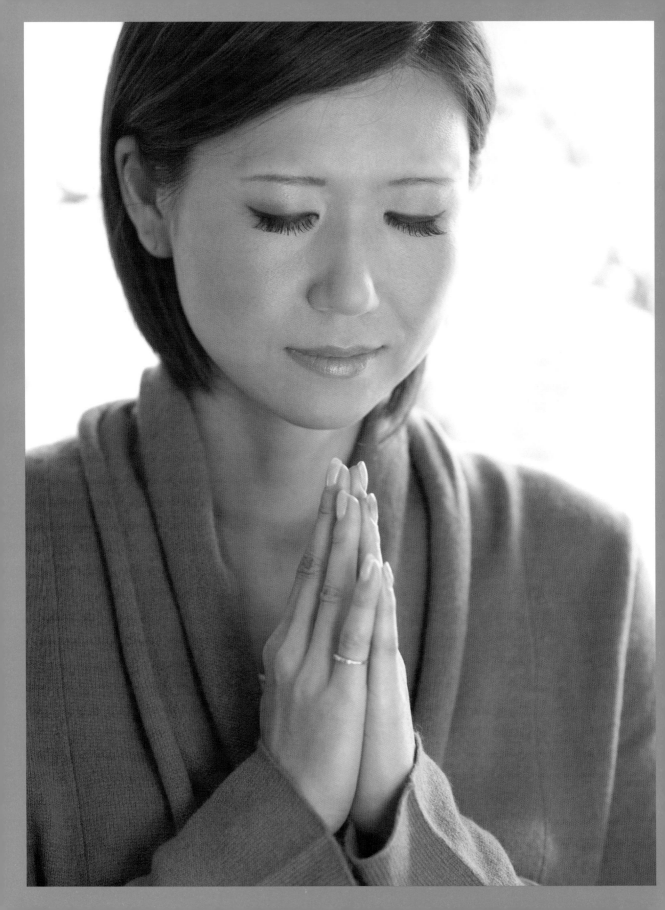

CHAPTER 3

The Emotional Connection

What do emotions have to do with skin? In my opinion, everything. Our skin can easily betray what's going on in our hearts and minds.

Since it's our largest and only visible organ, we often notice the effects of our feelings in our skin before anywhere else in our bodies. You need to be aware that emotional uproar can really do a number on your face. Not only does it age you, but it can contribute to acne, eczema, inflammation, and infection as well.

The aches and pain you experience as a result of stress can also be reflected in your face. And the disrupted sleep that tends to accompany tension and anxiety can further contribute to a sallow complexion and dark circles under your eyes.

Ever since I was a kid, my emotions have manifested in my skin issues—and I was reminded of that this past holiday season. When I was a child, Christmas wasn't about love and gift giving; it was more about emotional turmoil. The holidays were so stressful that I'd want to just crawl away and disappear for days.

Now I have a family of my own, including a young son, and I live in a beautiful home. Although I have nothing to complain about these days, I still have a hard time during the holidays. So leading up to Christmas one year, I was uptight, grumpy, and on edge. My stomach hurt, my back went out, one year my eczema flared, and I broke out in blemishes along my jawline. Those negative emotions needed to get out. And this was how they were doing it.

My solution was to go to my wonderful bodyworker, Mary. She got to work and massaged my muscles with her special technique, and tears suddenly began to roll down my face. Her expert manipulation released the energy my body was storing. I emerged a different person: my back was better, and my skin started to clear up. I always tell my clients to find where they're storing that pent-up negative energy and then look for ways to work it out of the body.

The Facialist Will See You Now

After so many years spent working with other people, I've developed an intuition and instinct about others' emotional states. I can touch someone and say, "Okay, what's going on?" I'm not psychic, but I can detect when there is pain in someone—when I'm in tune with my client, I can feel what she feels.

For example, one woman came into my clinic with the worst cystic acne I've ever seen in my life. She was so congested that every single pore had become infected, and she had terrible scarring as well. She came to me after a doctor had put her on a cocktail of topical and internal drugs. My team and I got her off the medications; and with treatments, products, and lifestyle changes, we cleared her skin in three months. But after some time, another cystic infection emerged on her lower cheek. We were both concerned because this wasn't your average kind of acne.

I sat her down and said, "Let's talk." It took a while, but I finally found out what was going on with her. It turned out her job had been really stressful because there was someone she didn't get along with, and this had brought up other issues in her life. My client ended up quitting her job, and her acne immediately went away. This is an example of how I teach my clients to connect the dots and figure out the issues that might be triggering their skin problems.

Many times during my career, facials have doubled as therapy sessions—for my clients and for me. Looking back, I can see that one of the reasons I immediately felt so at home in this profession was because it was like a healthy home came *to me*. Many of my clients were older ladies around my mom's age, and since I didn't have a functioning mother to actively support my life and my growth, these women played that role. We developed close, meaningful relationships: they encouraged and supported me—like my own mother never could—and I nurtured them, both by caring for their skin and helping to restore their confidence and sense of self through my touch and treatments. I could never help my mom, but I could help these ladies. It's almost like I've had hundreds of mothers over the years! And some of these women have followed me throughout my career and have stuck by my side. (One of them, Martha Kramer, is a very special client who actually helped me buy my first laser.)

If I've learned anything over the years, it's this: *We have to take time for ourselves.* If we constantly do things for others and never focus on ourselves, it will tear us down. I have a friend who's a marriage counselor, and she reinforced something that I instinctively knew. She said, "Take care of yourself first—make sure your spirit is healthy. Next, make sure that your relationship with your spouse is healthy. Then you can take care of your children." It's not so much an "order of importance," it's simply a formula that seems to be true because harmony results. If we don't love ourselves, we won't be happy, and that will affect our relationships. If we're arguing constantly with our spouse, the children feel it, and it will be very painful for them. I know—I've been the little girl on the other side of those arguments.

This message was brought home to me recently. Every morning I read a meditation to prepare myself for the day (I really like author Melody Beattie's meditations), and on this particular morning, the one I read was about nurturing yourself. There I was, lying in bed, anticipating a really hectic day with my seven-year-old. I'd promised to take him skiing, and I was worried. My son skis fast, and I'm nervous with him sometimes. I didn't think I could keep up; plus, as a mom, I wanted to keep him safe. Not to mention the fact that I was exhausted and wanted to just lie in bed. So I said to myself, *Katie, let's find a way to relax and enjoy this time.* I decided to take a long, luxurious shower; give myself a hair mask; and put on some makeup before we hit the slopes. Just doing those little things made me much more patient with my son. I was able to nurture him because I had taken the time to nurture myself.

I heard a story from a friend about a college professor who was famous for her over-the-top jewelry: She wore rings on every finger, necklaces, bangles, you name it! It was an affectionate joke around the university that her students knew she was approaching because she jingled. So when she stopped jingling, they knew that something was wrong. It turns out that the professor was going through some very serious family problems; while her students didn't know that, they did know that when she stopped wearing her jewelry, something was not right

Look out for your own clues. Are you keeping up with your personal grooming? Do you take care of your skin, hair, and nails? Do you take pride in putting yourself together, or does it feel like a chore? If the answer to any of these questions is no, you might want to do a little self-examination and see what's *really* going on in your life.

Reflecting on yourself can be a vicious cycle. Because when you don't feel good and you don't take care of yourself, it shows. And if you look in the mirror and don't like what you see, that *will* affect the way you do your job and treat your family, as well as how you feel. My client Lisa Rinna talks a lot about this in her book, *Rinnavation*. Taking the time to treat yourself impacts every part of your life. You might feel a little selfish, but those extra moments will color your whole attitude in a positive way. When you feel better about yourself, you will perform every role in your life better!

Of course not every skin problem is caused by how you're feeling about yourself or your mental state. Sometimes an issue is just an issue: it might be hormonal or because you're genetically predisposed to it. But do watch your skin. If you're having problems, ask yourself, "Where am I mentally and emotionally?" You might be getting a sign that it's time to make a change in your life.

I have so many stories that support this point—but the truth is, so does a lot of research. Emotions have a huge impact on your skin, and there is hard scientific evidence to back up the idea. Here are just some of the studies that have been done on the subject:

1. Researchers in Germany discovered that when children went through a traumatic event such as their parents' divorce, a death in the family, or a severe illness before age 14, they had a much higher chance of suffering from eczema.

2. A study funded by the Estée Lauder company, which focused on women going through stressful divorces, showed that their skin recovered much more slowly after injury than skin belonging to women who said that they were happy.

3. The *American Journal of Pathology* reported that stress activates the skin's immune cells, leading to inflammatory conditions such as dermatitis and psoriasis.

4. A study conducted by the Stanford University School of Medicine showed that the stress of exams caused students' acne to flare up, and that the more stressed the students reported being, the worse the effect on their skin. This has been reinforced by several other studies conducted around the world.

5. In a Japanese study of 26 people with dermatitis, their symptoms got better for two hours after watching a funny movie, even when they were exposed to the allergen that usually triggered their condition. It's believed that laughing reduced their levels of stress hormones.

6. Psoriasis patients who practiced meditation-based relaxation while having ultraviolet (UV) light treatments experienced faster clearing of their skin than those who received the light treatments alone, according to the results of a trial held at the University of Massachusetts Medical School.

7. In a Yale University study, people with melanoma, the deadliest form of skin cancer, were more likely to have lived through a stressful experience during the years leading up to their diagnosis than people who did not have skin cancer. Another study at Johns Hopkins University showed that mice exposed to fox urine (which stressed them out) got skin cancer much more quickly when put under UV rays than mice who weren't exposed.

The common denominator here is stress hormones and how they affect our immune system. Researchers have known for some time that stress impacts our ability to fight infections and stay healthy. Acute stress protects us from dangerous situations by stimulating our "fight or flight" response, which temporarily boosts our immune system to deal with whatever is challenging us. That kind of pressure is situational and is relieved when we take care of what's causing it.

Chronic stress is another matter altogether. This is when you're in a constant state of anxiety or fear over ongoing problems such as debt, a negative work situation, illness, an unhappy relationship, loneliness, or just a combination of factors that make up a modern crazy lifestyle. When you're suffering from chronic stress, you're existing in a constant "state of emergency," and your body was not meant to live that way. The continual strain actually depresses your immune system, causing your levels of stress hormones such as adrenaline and cortisol to stay high in your body. Consequently, you develop symptoms such as headaches, backaches, or an upset stomach and you have trouble sleeping. On top of that, when you're anxious or depressed you don't tend to eat properly (or digest the food you do eat) or get enough exercise.

For many of us, chronic stress accumulates in skin problems. Whether we're talking about eczema, acne, or premature aging, we stand a much better chance of keeping them under control if our immune system is functioning strongly.

Stress Less

None of us lives a completely stress-free existence. Life would be very bland if we didn't have a little bit of pressure every now and then to motivate and stimulate us. I also want to make the point that we don't have to be unhappy to be stressed. My family life is very fulfilling, and I have a lot of great things happening in my career; nevertheless, I'm often totally stressed-out by trying to keep a lot of balls in the air at the same time. Going on QVC with my skin-care collection is especially nerve-wracking. I love doing it, but there is so much pressure to ensure that we're giving out the right information, that I'm connecting with the viewers and helping them with their skin issues. And it's all live and nonstop. Think about that!

So dealing with stress should be part of your skin-care regimen. There are lots of effective ways to help relieve tension; some of you will respond better to one option than another, which is why I'm giving you several of them to try. Even if you *still* doubt that your emotions have anything to do with your skin, you'll become a believer after you see the positive results of getting into a regular stress-busting routine.

Try out one or more of the following suggestions, and then enjoy the "beauty bonus" that results.

1. PACED BREATHING

If you're feeling anxious, you may be breathing fast and shallowly or even holding your breath altogether. Get into the habit of stopping for a few minutes to concentrate on taking slow, deep breaths; it's a no-fail way to calm both your body and your mind.

Sit quietly somewhere and just become conscious of how you're breathing. The idea is to slow down to about 5 or 6 breaths a minute (the usual is about 15). Inhale deeply, using your diaphragm and pushing out your abdomen. Hold it for a few counts (but not so long that it makes you dizzy), and then very slowly let out the air. Studies have shown that this kind of breathing lowers your blood pressure and is beneficial to your health in many other ways—not the least of which is that it stimulates the flow of lymphatic fluid through your body, which in turn boosts your immune system.

I use this method before my QVC shows. Along with deep breathing, I do a visualization in which I picture the world. Then, when I'm looking into the camera, I imagine sending out a cloud of love and protection to surround the planet. And I have to tell you, there were times at QVC when I was so nervous because I knew that on live TV you can't make a mistake and you have to perform. But once I discovered this technique, it really helped calm me.

Beauty bonus: As well as getting you to relax, deep breathing affects blood circulation and the oxygenation of your cells, including those in your skin. And all cells need a steady stream of oxygen to keep them alive, deliver nutrition, and do their job properly.

2. PROGRESSIVE RELAXATION

Do you feel like you carry tension in your neck and shoulders? If so, you'll be happy to discover progressive relaxation, which is a great way to relieve muscle tension caused by stress.

Take off your shoes and loosen any tight clothing. Lie flat on the floor with your feet slightly apart and your arms by your sides, palms up. Cover yourself with a cozy blanket, if you like.

Become conscious of your breath. As you inhale, scrunch up a set of muscles as tightly as you can for about ten seconds, starting with your feet. Then, while you exhale, consciously let those muscles go—just let them flop. You're going to work your way up your body like this: legs, buttocks, stomach, chest, hands, arms, shoulders, neck, and face (including your tongue), clenching or stretching and then releasing. Allow all the tension to just melt away . . . until your entire body feels heavy, relaxed, and supported by the floor. You might even drift off to sleep, but do try to stay awake until you've worked your way through your entire body.

Once you become familiar with how relaxed muscles feel, you'll be able to release them throughout the day whenever you become aware that you're tensing up.

Beauty bonus: There are dozens of small muscles in the face, and it's one of the places we hold tension without realizing it. Notice if *your* face is tensed up at night, even as your head hits the pillow. Only when you consciously relax those muscles around your eyes, mouth, and jaw will you become aware of how you're contributing to the formation of wrinkles.

3. MEDITATION

I became convinced about the power of meditation after I witnessed significant changes in the skin of several of my clients who practice it. It really made me aware that I may be able to help someone topically or assist her in altering her diet, but if I can't help her find a way to stop her brain craziness, she's simply not going to look her best.

Meditation is a state of deep physical relaxation combined with acute mental alertness, and there are many ways to achieve this state. Almost every religion incorporates meditative practices such as praying or chanting, and you might be able to find one in your belief system. Other purely physiological techniques involve sitting and focusing on something that will hold your attention: a word, an image, your breath, or a visual cue.

Find a place to sit where you won't be disturbed for anywhere from 5 to 30 minutes. You don't have to sit cross-legged on the floor unless you want to. It's perfectly fine to sit in a straight-backed chair with your feet flat on the ground and your hands resting in your lap.

Close your eyes. Breathe easily and naturally, but focus on the feeling of your breath entering and leaving your body: notice how it feels cool as you breathe in and warm as you breathe out. As you relax, start to silently say a word as you exhale. It can be anything that's meaningful to you; many people repeat peaceful words such as *love* or simply *one.* You can also meditate on something visual: your child's face, a flower, the ocean, or anything that makes you feel happy and serene.

The idea here is to clear your head of your inner chatter. It's impossible to make your mind empty, of course, but if you find yourself dwelling on the subjects that stress you out, bring your attention back to your breath and the word you're saying or the image you're visualizing.

Meditating is most effective as a stress reliever when you do it regularly, so try to carve out a few minutes every day for your practice. I know that it's not always easy to meditate at first, which is why a great tool to help you get started is a guided-meditation CD. A couple you might find helpful are *The Beginner's Guide to Meditation* by Joan Z. Borysenko, Ph.D., and *Meditations for Overcoming Life's Stresses and Strains* by Bernie S. Siegel, M.D.

Beauty bonus: Meditation causes stress hormones in your blood to drop and boosts your immune system.

4. YOGA

Like meditation, yoga is another ancient practice that's a terrific stress buster for our modern times and is credited with any number of health and psychological benefits. The whole yoga scene can be a bit confusing, however, as there are so many different kinds available now. It can be soothing if you choose one that's oriented toward flexibility and stretching, or what you'll often hear called "restorative yoga." Or it can be more energizing if you go with a flow-and-strength approach that challenges your heart and muscles—if this appeals to you, then power yoga would be the way to go. Some types of yoga are strictly physical, while others have a spiritual component; many also incorporate breathing exercises.

Telling you how to do yoga is outside the scope of this book, but it's so popular that you're sure to find a class near you. If you prefer to practice alone, however, there are hundreds of books, CDs, and DVDs on the market where you can find instruction. Whether you take a class or pursue yoga on your own, be sure to look into the different types so that you find the method that works best for relieving your stress.

Beauty bonus: Classical hatha yoga (as opposed to other more rigorous forms and the hybrid classes that are popular now) was studied at Jefferson Medical College in Philadelphia and found to reduce cortisol levels, which, as you now know, contribute to unhealthy skin.

I'd also like to add that many of my celebrity clients are yoga fanatics. I can always identify them because they have that "yoga body"—a lean, balanced, graceful look that's a definite beauty bonus.

5. EXERCISE

Exercise, particularly cardio (that is, the kind that makes your heart really pump) is known to help relieve stress, boost spirits, fight symptoms of depression, and increase your brain's production of those feel-good endorphins. Endorphins are responsible for what's known as the "runner's high," but any vigorous activity promotes this same response, be it cycling, dancing, swimming, or playing sports.

Not all exercise needs to be strenuous, however—something like a 30-minute walk, especially outdoors, can give you a very healthy payoff. In fact, when I see people in my clinic who are clearly in a funk and can't seem to muster the energy to get out of it, I always say that the best thing is to go for a walk. That alone can change how you feel about yourself.

I try to exercise every morning. Like deep breathing, I know that physical activity also helps my lymphatic fluid get moving through my body, sweeping out cellular debris and toxins and boosting my immune system.

Beauty bonus: Exercise does more than just lift your spirits. It gets your blood flowing and increases oxygen flow throughout your body, including to your skin. Researchers have recently found a direct link between moderate exercise and decreased inflammation of damaged skin tissue, and they think that it might have something to do with this increased blood and oxygen. Studies also show that the skin of those who exercise is physically thicker than those who don't.

6. SWEAT

Exercising really hard is certainly one way to work up a sweat, but I believe that sweating in general is amazing. When you're in a sauna, steam room, or hot tub (my personal favorite) and your body gets to that elevated heat level, it releases emotional pain from your body. Of course, it also helps with physical aches and pains and the stiff muscles that result from a stressful lifestyle.

I don't believe it's by chance that so many cultures have some kind of "sweat bath" tradition: from hammams ("Turkish baths") to sweat lodges, people all around the world and all throughout time have enjoyed the benefits of steaming toxins from the skin. Ayurveda—the ancient Indian healing tradition—alone uses 13 ways to make you sweat!

Just be sure to stay hydrated when you practice this stress buster; that is, drink plenty of water to replace what you're losing. If exercise gives you shortness of breath or chest pains, then stay away from excessive heat sources. I also recommend that you avoid the Scandinavian practice of going from heat to a cold shower. And pregnant women should forgo saunas, steam rooms, and hot tubs, especially in their first trimester.

Beauty bonus: Steam is a basic component of a facial because it opens your pores and helps with cleansing. Heat also relaxes blood vessels and improves circulation.

7. MASSAGE

I've already told you how bodywork has helped me deal with the traumatic events I hold in my body—I recommend finding a good bodyworker to everyone. The most commonly available type of bodywork is massage, and you don't have to be a scientist to know that getting one of these is a great way to get rid of stress. But massage has also been shown to reduce anxiety, elevate mood, ease pain, lower blood pressure, and be helpful with insomnia. It seems to promote the release of the brain's natural opiates, which encourages a feeling of well-being. Add in restful music and aromatherapy—particularly when you use calming essential oils, such as lavender, neroli, and sandalwood—and you get extra benefits.

There are a number of different types of massage. Just as with yoga, there are some that are gentle and relaxing and others that are more vigorous. Swedish massage is the one you're most likely to run across, and it's a good one to try if you're new to the idea because it's soothing and gentle. Deep-tissue massage targets deeper layers of muscle and connective tissue and can be quite intense. Yet there are any number of styles in between, such as Shiatsu, Thai, reflexology (which targets your feet), and hot stone. There are even specific massages for athletes, pregnant women, and the elderly.

If you want to experiment with different styles to find the one that de-stresses you the most, see if there is a massage-therapy school in your area—they often want volunteers for students to practice on. And if you've never experienced a massage because you feel a bit uncomfortable about the idea of undressing and lying naked under a sheet while a stranger touches you, break yourself in with a 10- or 15-minute neck-and-shoulder massage. These are increasingly available all over the place. Once you become aware of how amazing massage can be, you'll be hooked.

Beauty bonus: Massage can also help to promote lymphatic drainage. As I mentioned previously, your lymphatic system is a complex network of vessels, ducts, and organs that is responsible for moving toxins away from healthy cells. Massage aids in moving the fluid through that system, helping eliminate metabolic waste, excess fluid, and bacteria. Lymphatic massage also assists in hydrating your skin, dispersing toxins, and clearing up acne; and it may even improve the appearance of cellulite.

The Beauty of Balance

Building a multifaceted business such as mine can be very challenging, even though I enjoy it. As I've gone down this professional skin-care path, I've encountered my fair share of obstacles and dead ends. When I've come up against a wall, sometimes it's taken me down and I've been crushed; other times I've just thought, *Oh, wrong way.* But every single time I've learned something.

I believe that if you're blocked, it's most often because you're supposed to look in another direction, so go another way. Life is almost like a maze, and when you don't know which way to go or what path to choose, try what I do: look to your higher power for guidance and direction.

When you pray or meditate or are just quiet in nature, life will come to be more balanced. When you're not balanced, you tend to be locked in that survival mode. I've had some huge decisions to make recently, personally and professionally. And getting quiet was the only way I was able to come to the right ones. Eckhart Tolle's book *The Power of Now* has had a big influence on me. I used to react to every thought I had, be it positive or negative. I'd go in all different directions and make hasty decisions, changing my mind often. Once I became aware of my behavior, I realized I could sit on a feeling and wait for a decision. I now encourage my clients to find their present moment and their state of balance, since balance will always benefit the skin.

And that brings us to the next chapter. A balanced and complexion-friendly diet is a necessary element to gorgeous skin. It's an important part of the Skin Health Pyramid, and when applied, can make all the difference in the world . . . not only affecting your skin, but also your entire state of mind.

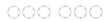

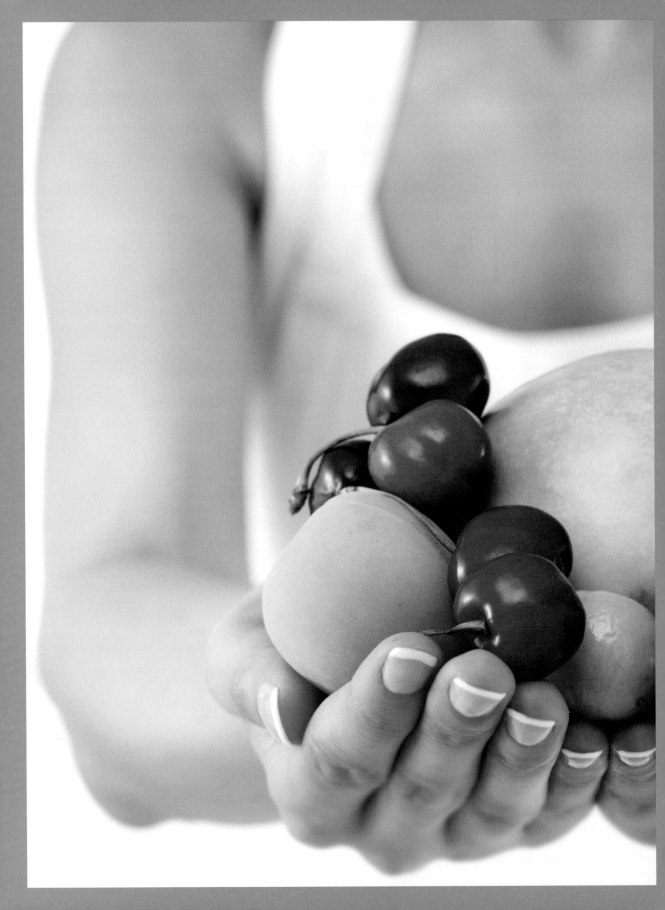

CHAPTER 4

Beauty and the Buffet

I have always been an athlete. Growing up, I ran track and was the fastest sprinter at my high school. I've always felt more at home on a hike or on horseback than at a fancy party in a pair of high heels. When I was young, we'd take weekend trips into the Sierra Nevada mountains, weaving our way through what my dad calls "the backcountry." In my opinion, the Sierras contain some of the most beautiful places on Earth. My husband, son, and I continue to go there every once in a while, and I find it so rewarding.

To this day, I prefer the outdoors to the indoors so much that virtually every car I've owned has been a convertible!

Challenging my body, muscles, stamina, and physical strength has never been the issue. However, the other key to healthy skin and a healthy lifestyle *has* been: *diet*. And for me, I'm usually all-or-nothing. Either I'm eating healthy, clean, nutritious, and organic—or I'm totally off the wagon. The buffet is my weakness.

Everyone knows the expression "You are what you eat." Well, if that's the case, then most of the time I'm a burrito! I love Mexican food, and if I've had a hard day or I'm feeling down, I get on the phone and place an order to go. Despite everything I've learned and seen over the years, food has always been my place of refuge—so when the going gets a little tough, I get out the chips and salsa!

I really wish I could tell you that I eat the perfect diet for my skin all the time. I do my best, but like so many women today, I'm juggling a career and family responsibilities. And in my case, I also travel a lot, so I'm constantly eating in airports and hotels or just grabbing whatever is available. When I'm home and have the time, I get back on track and make the effort to cook and eat healthfully and make better choices. I can always see the difference in how I look and feel.

Yet even though I've always known the power a healthy diet has on the state and shape of the body, I didn't truly understand the dramatic difference such a diet could have on the skin until I witnessed it firsthand. Someone I love very much overhauled his diet and, in turn, got a new lease on life—and on his skin!

The Acid Test: Alkaline Versus Acidic

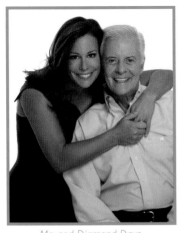

Me and Diamond Dave.

Seven years ago my father-in-law, Dave Somerville, was diagnosed with stage 5 prostate cancer. The lead singer of the 1950s group the Diamonds, "Diamond Dave," as he is known by his fans, was still performing his hits, such as "Little Darlin'" (my favorite!) and "Why Do Fools Fall in Love?" all over the country. A truly inspirational man, he immediately took action and began to research his options. He was determined to find the best possible solution and get back on the road.

Four different doctors presented treatment options such as surgery and radiation, but Dave decided to go with a different approach. He'd always been interested in nutrition and alternative health, and when a friend recommended a naturopathic doctor in San Diego, he found what he was looking for: a doctor who "laughs at cancer." I was nervous; in fact, I honestly thought at first that it was a mistake. Yet this is where I first learned how dramatically nutrition can impact the skin.

Dave's treatment regimen focused on organic foods, a range of immunity-boosting supplements, and drinking nothing but purified water—lots of it. Most important, he maintained an alkaline environment in his body, the basis of his naturopathic doctor's protocol. Dave ate foods that alkalized his body and minimized those that acidified it, helping maintain his body in a healthy pH range and reducing disease-causing acid waste in his system. The theory (one not supported by the traditional medical community) is that cancer cells don't grow in an alkaline environment.

My father-in-law was completely committed to this program, and in less than a year's time, his cancer disappeared. Total recovery. I know this sounds unbelievable, but the strategy miraculously worked for him. I'm telling you this story here in this book because of the *other* changes I saw—changes in his *skin*. I couldn't believe it, but I actually saw brown spots and sun damage disappear from Dave's face, in the same way that the cancer vanished. From a clinician's perspective, I thought, *This is impossible.* I'd never seen anything like it in my life. Generally, when people in my line of work see sun spots and pigment issues, we treat them with topical peels, usually aggressively, and topical products. I was blown away, because Dave's skin glowed. I mean, it literally *glowed.* To this day, he stays very close to the parameters of the diet, and looks a decade younger than his actual years.

To be sure, the choices my father-in-law made were fairly extreme, and he was absolutely dedicated to the strategy. However, I cannot deny the impact that this diet had on his health and his appearance. Since his recovery, I've made my own commitment to eating a healthier diet, whenever I can. Like I said, food is my weak point, but I'm more aware than ever before of the power, both positive and negative, that my food choices make on my skin. And what's even more powerful is that I get to share this story with my clients, and it's become part of my professional tool kit. I know that if certain clients are experiencing extremely challenging skin issues, lifestyle changes have to be made to get the results we desire.

The Organic Choice

Our food today is simply not as nutrient rich as it was 50 years ago. Industrialized, conventional farming has impacted the nutritional value of what we eat. So has the emergence of boxed and processed foods, not to mention the contemporary ways we raise our poultry and cattle. Everything my father-in-law ate was organic because he needed all of the vitamins, minerals, amino acids, and antioxidants he could get to fight off the intruder in his body. Organically grown fruits and vegetables have been proven time and time again to have higher levels of antioxidants, proteins, and nutrients necessary for our bodies to function efficiently. In fact, antioxidant levels have been found to be 30 percent higher on average than those found in conventionally grown produce.

Meat is not that different. Because of the increased demand for beef and poultry, aka our "fast-food nation," farms raising these animals resort to questionable strategies. Many are fed foods that aren't natural to their constitution to fatten them up as fast as possible, along with hormones to make them grow bigger. If you've ever had organically raised, grass-fed beef, you can tell the difference. My dad, who raises this kind of beef, simply has to take a look at it to do so—noting that the color and texture are different, as is the smell.

These unnatural hormones in our food can disrupt our own hormones and throw them out of balance, causing all kinds of issues, including skin disorders. I'm certain that the excess hormones in our dairy products and meats have contributed to the increase in the occurrence of acne in recent decades. There are studies that support this belief, which I'll touch upon a little later.

For me, a healthy diet is about healthy choices (most of the time!) and moderation. And for the majority of us, the best way to encourage health and well-being—which will always show up in our skin—is to eat more vegetables and fruits and less saturated fat, sugar, white flour, and packaged foods. But because I'm not an expert nutritionist, I asked my colleague and friend Dr. David Rahm to help me summarize the most important stuff for you.

Dr. Rahm and the 80/20 Rule

Along with my father-in-law, Dr. Rahm heightened my awareness and commitment to health and nutrition. We first met and worked together at a cosmetic-surgery practice in Southern California years ago, before I opened my clinic on Melrose Place.

This large practice gave clients a progressive, integrative approach to age management: the surgeons administrated cosmetic surgery, Dr. Rahm offered wellness and nutritional counseling, and I provided professional skin-care treatments.

Shortly after I met David, he launched an incredibly innovative line of skin health supplements and was the first doctor I know of to do so. He asked my advice when formulating the line, and I gave him my suggestions based on what my clients needed. His company, VitaMedica, formulates and develops the highest-quality, whole-food supplements on the market in a variety of categories: from those that help support skin that's mature, acne prone, or recovering from surgery, to those that provide everyday nutritional needs. In 2008, a dream came true when we worked together to create the Kate Somerville/VitaMedica collection of skin health supplements, now a powerful and effective weapon in my arsenal to fight aging and acne. Because Dr. Rahm knows more about health and wellness (and any other topic you can think of) than anyone I know, naturally I asked him to help me with this chapter, and to share his best advice for what he so often calls wellness and "age management."

Dr. Rahm's first healthy diet commandment is what he calls the "80/20" rule. That means you eat your healthy best 80 percent of the time, and then allow for foods that aren't so great (but you really enjoy) the other 20 percent. For some, this might mean that you'll have healthy food during the week and indulge on the weekend (this is what I try to do). Like anything, it requires discipline and effort, but everything that's worthwhile requires a little hard work! What I usually find is that once I get on a roll of eating nutritiously, I start to crave sweets and junk less and less. This will happen to you, too—your taste buds will recalibrate, and before long, sweets will be too sweet, simple carbs will be too heavy, and you'll be craving the healthy stuff! While radiant skin is the goal of this book, your entire body will benefit from a better diet: a fitter figure, increased energy, and improved brain function will almost always result.

The Skin Health Diet

Per Dr. Rahm's orders, I try to eat foods that contain ample lean protein, plenty of low-glycemic-load carbohydrates (nonstarchy vegetables and fruits), and moderate amounts of beneficial fat. The key is to eat high-quality, nutrient-dense foods on a daily basis.

Let's talk specifics now. What follows are a few guidelines Dr. Rahm gave me to help you select foods from the three macronutrient categories—carbohydrates, protein, and fat—that promote skin health.

1. COMPLEX OR "SLOW" CARBS

You've heard it a million times: eat a range of differently colored fruits and vegetables. That's because they provide an excellent source of vitamins, minerals, phytonutrients, antioxidants, and fiber. Those gorgeous, glossy fruits and veggies that are deep blue, purple, or red (such as blueberries and raspberries) have higher levels of protective compounds called polyphenols and are very high in antioxidants.

But there's another, slightly more complicated reason why you should add more produce to your plate. Most of these natural, healthy foods have a very low glycemic index (GI), which keeps the body in balance. In contrast, high GI foods include a lot of processed and packaged items like candy, cookies, soft drinks, baked goods, and other nutritionally deficient foods. The GI indicates the effects of carbohydrates on blood glucose and corresponding insulin levels, which can have many effects on your health. When it comes to skin, however, research conducted by Loren Cordain, Ph.D., the author of *The Paleo Diet,* has shown that heightened insulin levels (caused by eating high GI foods) starts a hormonal cascade that can result in myriad issues, including . . . breakouts!

Other research shows that good nutrition actually keeps wrinkles at bay. For example, a study done in Australia discovered that older people who ate a lot of vegetables, legumes, and olive oil had less wrinkling and aging in areas exposed to the sun than those whose diet contained more meat, milk, butter or margarine, and sugar. Yep—that is exactly why "Diamond Dave" Somerville glows. He practically drinks shots of olive oil!

To get our GI down, most of us have got to add in more fruits and vegetables— even if we eat out as often as I do. If you're at a restaurant for breakfast, ask for sliced tomatoes or fresh fruit instead of home fries or hash browns. For lunch, opt for the salad instead of a burger. For dinner, replace potatoes, rice, or pasta with additional green vegetables. Start replacing potato chips with baby carrots. And for dessert, eat a bowl of fresh berries and accent with a bit of dark chocolate.

2. HIGH-QUALITY LEAN PROTEIN

The building blocks of protein—amino acids—are important for the skin because they're needed to develop collagen and elastin. They're especially important if you're having treatments or using topical ingredients that promote exfoliation and skin-cell turnover.

Over the years, red meat has become the bad guy of nutrition because it's associated with so many health issues. But it turns out that meat itself isn't necessarily the real problem—rather, it's the saturated fat in the meat. Beef, poultry, ham, and even farm-raised fish are fattened quickly so that they can be processed and sold. This causes the meat to contain much higher amounts of total and saturated fat, which is not beneficial to our general health or our skin. In addition, these "factory farmed" animals are often fed antibiotics and hormones that are then passed on to us when we eat the meat. While this isn't good for anyone, it's even more problematic for those of us with acne-prone skin.

Still, we really need to eat lean, high-quality protein. The key is to look for grass-fed beef, free-range chicken or turkey, and wild-caught fish because they're lower in saturated and total fat and have more of the beneficial omega-3 fatty acids that we've come to associate with good skin. If you can't find these in your local grocery store, search out producers and ranchers who offer their high-quality meats on the Internet. I promise you will taste the difference.

Look for organic eggs reinforced with DHA (docosahexaenoic acid), which is a beneficial omega-3 fatty acid. Keep in mind that yogurt provides not only protein but calcium and beneficial bacteria. However, be sure to look for organic brands that are free of additives and hormones; in addition, buy low- or nonfat plain yogurt and add your own fruit. Beans are also a good source of protein and fiber and can be added to soups, stews, and salads.

3. HIGH-QUALITY, UNSATURATED FATS

I'm sure you've heard that you should replace saturated fats, trans fats, and partially hydrogenated fats with health-promoting omega-3 fatty acids. While your body also needs omega-6, our modern diet tends to contain an overabundance of it, causing an imbalance in the ratio of omega-6 to omega-3. This imbalance promotes inflammation, which influences skin health because it can cause skin cells to stick together, blocking pores and leading to breakouts. Boost your intake of omega-3s and reduce inflammation by eating fish such as albacore tuna, mackerel, salmon, herring, and sardines once or twice a week.

Adding raw, unsalted nuts to salads and fruits is also a great way to boost the nutrition of any meal. Walnuts especially provide an excellent source of the essential omega-3 fatty acid called alpha-linolenic acid. This fat is very important for building cell membranes, which is a significant consideration when you understand that skin cells turn over more rapidly than most other cells in the body.

Olive oil is an excellent source of monounsaturated fat that's ideal for use in salad dressings and in most cooking. When buying olive oil, you want to look for "extra virgin" on the label, which denotes that it's taken from the first pressing of the olives, has no chemical additives, and is not mixed with any other oil. Olive oil also serves as an incredible skin hydrator. Stock up on the stuff and you can safely use it all over your skin—it works great as an after-shower moisturizer to lock in hydration!

Complexion Cuisine

As you can see, feeding our skin from within is not that complicated. We just have to commit to taking better care of our bodies and respecting all the work they do for us. The overall goal is to eat a wide variety of fresh, healthy foods, in order to obtain the breadth and depth of the nutrients we need. But there are some foods that are powerhouses of nutrition, and you should try to fit them into your diet on a regular basis. While you've probably read about most of these, it's always nice to be reminded of the staples that we should put on the grocery list.

Here are my top 15 favorites when it comes to cooking for your complexion:

1. Almonds. A one-ounce serving (about 20 nuts) is an excellent source of vitamin E and magnesium, as well as a good source of copper, riboflavin, and fiber. Almonds also have monounsaturated fat and small amounts of protein, potassium, calcium, and iron. Researchers have found that the main bioflavonoids (plant-based compounds) in almonds provide the highest degree of antioxidant protection out there. Like most nuts, I recommend eating them raw and unsalted. And while almond milk doesn't quite pack the same nutritional punch, it does provide a great alternative to cow's milk for cereals and smoothies. (Be sure to look for unsweetened brands.)

Want to change it up a bit? Try walnuts, Brazil nuts, hazelnuts, or cashews. Most nuts are a great source of B vitamins, and the healthy fats in them benefit your skin's collagen.

2. Avocados. Containing nearly 20 vitamins, minerals, and phytonutrients—including vitamins C, B_9 (folate), and E; not to mention iron, potassium, lutein, and beta-carotene—avocados are also what are known as a "nutrient booster." That's because they enhance the absorption of fat-soluble nutrients, such as carotenes, in foods that you eat with them. They also provide fiber and are rich in healthy mono- and polyunsaturated fat. These fats make avocados very luscious and satisfying to eat (but also calorific; just a quarter of one is a serving). Slice avocados on salad, spread them on bread as a butter or mayo substitute, and mash them into guacamole dip (my preferred way!).

3. Black beans. All beans are packed with antioxidants, but studies have found that the darker the bean, the more it contains (makes sense—the same usually applies to veggies). A 3.5-ounce serving of black beans contains about ten times more antioxidants than the equivalent amount of oranges. In terms of antioxidant levels, black beans are followed by red, brown, yellow, and then white beans. And all beans are a great source of fiber.

4. Blueberries. I *love* blueberries and have them almost every morning in a smoothie. Despite their small size, studies have shown that compared with 20 other fruits, wild blueberries have the highest level of antioxidants per serving. Not only that, but they also fight inflammation at the cellular level, which is a significant factor in degenerative aging. High in fiber, they're also low on the glycemic index. One serving is about a half cup, and you can enjoy your berries on cereal or desserts or just eat them like candy. Try dried blueberries or blueberry juice, too.

Although blueberries top the nutritional charts, all berries—raspberries, strawberries, cranberries, blackberries—are right up there, so load up on them, be they fresh, frozen, or dried. But do keep in mind that fresh berries are among the foods you should definitely buy organic because they're often sprayed with pesticides.

5. Flaxseed. I've been sold on flaxseed since I introduced it into my own diet years ago. It's very high in omega-3s and may be a more acceptable way to get them if you aren't a big fan of fish. (That would be me!) Flaxseeds can be ground or extracted for their oil, which should never be heated but can be used on salads. You also can take the oil in capsule form.

When ground, flaxseeds provide an excellent source of both soluble and insoluble fiber—you can get whole flaxseeds that can be ground in a coffee or spice grinder as needed, or you can buy them already ground. With its nutty flavor, it's easy to add one to two tablespoons of ground flaxseed meal into cereal, sprinkle onto your salad, blend into a smoothie or yogurt, or bake it into muffins.

6. Green tea. Green tea has polyphenols (plant compounds) that seem to be better antioxidants than even vitamin C, and it has anti-inflammatory and anti-carcinogenic properties as well. Studies show that green tea can reduce the risk of damage from UV rays: the polyphenols don't block sunlight, but they can interfere with the chemical changes that could lead to the uncontrolled cell division typical of cancer. Green tea is also being studied as a possible new treatment for psoriasis and wound healing because one of its polyphenols seems to revive dying skin cells, at least in the laboratory.

It's the polyphenols that also give green tea its bitter flavor. While black tea is a more popular drink, it was believed that it lost its healthful properties in the drying process. However, newer studies have shown that black tea does have many of the same antioxidant properties as green tea. White tea—which is made from the young, delicate leaves of the tea bush—is still another option.

7. Melons. We're getting a "twofer" here as I'm grouping cantaloupe and watermelon together. Cantaloupe is an excellent source of vitamins A and C, making it an antioxidant dream, and it has folate and potassium. Watermelon is an outstanding source of the same antioxidants, getting its pink color from its concentration of lycopene, the cancer fighter that makes tomatoes so healthy. Both melons give you fiber and contribute to your daily intake of water because of their juiciness.

Eat this wonder fruit as is—what's better than a cool slab of melon on a hot day? You can also make fruit salads, juice it (but you'll lose the fiber), or even make melon soup.

8. Olive oil. Olive oil has been used topically as a beauty treatment since ancient times, but nutritionally speaking, this rich oil is also high in monounsaturated fat and is a good source of antioxidant polyphenols.

9. Pomegranate. Used as folk medicine since biblical times, pomegranates pack potent health benefits. Studies in Israel show that the fruit has more antioxidant properties than red wine and green tea. Pomegranates also provide isoflavones, potassium, vitamin C, and niacin. Eat the fruit or drink them juiced—the juice makes great smoothies and is even showing up in exotic cocktails (Pomegranate Cosmo, anyone?).

10. Wild salmon. Salmon is extremely rich in omega-3 fatty acids and can be baked, grilled, panfried, or poached. The key is to eat wild salmon fished from its natural environment, where it lives on krill and shrimp (which give it that pink color). Farmed salmon is fed fish meal laced with antibiotics and must be dyed pink—otherwise, it's a grayish color. Note that most canned salmon is wild and tends to come complete with bones, which are a great source of calcium. Canned salmon is excellent in salads or on sandwiches. (And be sure to experiment with other cold-water, fatty fish such as mackerel, sardines, herring, and rainbow trout.)

11. Spinach. This vegetable is a tremendous source of vitamins (B, C, and E); minerals (potassium, calcium, iron, and magnesium); and, this may surprise you, omega-3s. Many studies have shown that the carotenoids in spinach can slow down skin-cancer cells and protect against signs of aging.

Actually, spinach is here representing *all* of the dark green, leafy vegetables because it's the one most common in our diets. It's that dark green color that gives you a clue as to the heavy concentration of nutrients. The smartest thing you could do for yourself dietwise is to introduce a lot more of these greens into your daily menu because they all have slightly different groups of vitamins and phytonutrients. Collard, turnip, and dandelion greens; kale; chard; dark green cabbage; and the old standbys of broccoli and brussels sprouts can be steamed, cooked in soups or stews, stir-fried, or even finely chopped and eaten raw in salads.

12. Tomatoes. As I mentioned when I talked about melons, tomatoes are a rich source of lycopene, which is a potent antioxidant. Early and ongoing research suggests that lycopene reduces the risk of skin cancer. In fact, eating a sauce made by simmering tomatoes in olive oil has been shown to protect the skin from sunburns, about the same amount as using a sunblock with an SPF of two or three.

Your body more easily absorbs lycopene when tomatoes are processed into juice, sauce, or paste or when cooked—but, unfortunately, fried green tomatoes won't cut it. You see, it's the red color that denotes the presence of lycopene (watermelon and pink grapefruit also have smaller amounts of it).

13. Whole grains. By definition, whole grains contain all of the essential parts of the entire seed. They can be cracked, crushed, rolled, and cooked; but they cannot be refined, which means that they've had the bran, germ, and nutrients stripped away.

Whole grains have been widely studied for their health benefits. For example, doctors at Cornell University discovered that whole grains contain as much or more protective antioxidants than many fruits and vegetables—wheat and oats almost equal broccoli and spinach. Whole grains have also been found to be anti-inflammatory, and they provide you with loads of fiber. In addition, whole grains were a big part of an anti-acne diet formulated by researchers in Australia.

How exactly do we tie all of the suggestions in this chapter into a healthy lifestyle? Here is a sample menu of what you might eat on an average day to promote healthy skin:

Upon Waking

1 (8 oz.) glass of water with the juice of ½ lemon squeezed into it

Breakfast

1 serving of steel-cut oatmeal, sweetened with stevia

½ cup fresh or frozen blueberries or other fresh fruit in season

¼ cup walnut halves

2 cups nonfat, plain yogurt (try Greek-style yogurt for a tangy taste and creamy texture)

Midmorning Snack

1 slice of watermelon or cantaloupe

¼ cup unsalted almonds

1 cup of green tea

Lunch

A big green salad:

2 cups mixed dark leafy greens: spinach, romaine lettuce, finely chopped chard or kale, dandelion or beet leaves

¼ avocado, sliced

1 chopped tomato

1 sliced cucumber

1 sliced red pepper

¼ cup garbanzo beans or black beans

4 oz. organic chicken breast

Shredded carrot

Sliced scallion

Salad dressing including flaxseed oil and lemon juice

1 slice of whole-grain bread with olive oil for dipping

Midafternoon Snack

1 sliced apple

2 tablespoons natural peanut butter

1 cup of green tea

Dinner

4 oz. wild salmon

1 baked yam

Steamed broccoli and asparagus sprinkled with toasted pumpkin seeds

1 glass of red wine

Bedtime

1 cup of chamomile tea (or other soothing herbal tea of your choice)

You're probably most familiar with wheat, rice, oats, and rye. However, there is a whole world of other grains that you should try, including amaranth, quinoa, millet, and barley—all are really versatile grains. Try to replace your breakfast cereal in the morning with one of these new choices, add to a soup, or season and serve at dinner as a savory side dish.

14. Yams and sweet potatoes. It's beta-carotene, a precursor to vitamin A, that gives these vegetables their distinctive coloring: they're packed with it. They're also a good source of vitamins B_6 and C, copper, and potassium; and they add fiber to your diet. On top of that, they're also lower on the glycemic index than white potatoes, so they're less likely to cause inflammation.

We tend to think of these veggies as "holiday" food, but they're available all year. Roast them in olive oil, boil and mash them, or simply stick them in the microwave and zap them for about four minutes.

15. Yogurt. There's no denying that yogurt has many health benefits: if you stick to low- or nonfat varieties and avoid those with added sugar, you'll get protein, calcium, vitamins B_2 and B_{12}, potassium, and magnesium. Some brands are also fortified with vitamin D.

I'm not a huge fan of dairy, but I do enjoy yogurt because it has probiotics that help add healthy bacteria to the intestines. A study at the Human Nutrition Research Center on Aging at Tufts University in Boston showed that yogurt changes the microflora in the gastrointestinal tract, regulates the passage of food through the digestive system, and enhances the immune system.

You know, now that I think about it, you could easily make the Mexican food I love so much into a skin-healthy meal. Start with a taco: take a warm corn or whole-wheat tortilla and fill it with chicken breast, onions, and red peppers cooked in olive oil. Add a side of black beans and brown rice topped with salsa, guacamole, and plain yogurt instead of sour cream. If you like, you could even have it with a watermelon margarita! Perhaps you can take this as a challenge to turn your own favorite food into Complexion Cuisine.

Spices are powerhouses packed with antioxidant energy: some have even been found to have more antioxidant activity than fruits and veggies! For example, when comparing even weight of leaf to flesh, oregano has 42 times the antioxidant power of an apple (whoa!) and 4 times that of blueberries (wow!). Ginger helps digestion; clove is an anti-inflammatory; and cinnamon has been found to lower blood-sugar levels and kill bad bacteria from the inside. Always remember that as with most foods, the fresher the spice, the better for you and your skin. So sprinkle away!

Beauty-Busting Hit List

If the 15 foods I laid out on the previous pages nourish your skin, the next 5 do not. Instead, they promote inflammation and aging and may contribute to other issues, such as acne, eczema, rosacea, and psoriasis. Avoid the following whenever possible:

1. Refined white sugar and high-fructose corn syrup. Watch out for these two in prepackaged foods. Much of the sugar we get on a daily basis comes from beverages, so be careful what you drink, too. And don't be fooled by agave syrup and honey—yes, they're natural, but both contain simple sugars. Get your "sugar" rush from the herb stevia, now being marketed as a sweetener under the brand name Truvia.

2. Salt. Many packaged and processed foods are loaded with sodium—but so are the ones we think of as being healthier, like breakfast cereals. If you're waking up with puffy eyes every morning, you might want to take a look at your salt intake because it promotes edema or swelling. In addition, most salt is iodized, and iodine can exacerbate acne. When buying canned beans, either go for low-sodium brands or be sure to rinse them to remove sodium before eating.

3. Refined white flour and grain products. Replace with whole-wheat flour, whole-wheat pasta, and whole-grain baked goods. The nutrients haven't been stripped out of them and they provide more health benefits.

4. Trans fatty acids and hydrogenated or partially hydrogenated oils. These disease-promoting oils are found principally in packaged, processed foods. If you shift your diet toward more fruits and vegetables, you'll naturally reduce your intake of these unhealthy oils.

5. Saturated fat. This type of fat is solid at room temperature and is found in fatty meats and dairy products. Select lean cuts of meat, and be sure to remove the fat and skin. And stick to low- or nonfat dairy products—better yet, substitute cow's milk with almond, rice, or hemp milk.

✧✧✧

As a final note on beauty busters, I also recommend you limit your consumption of dairy, caffeine, and alcohol. While all do have some health-promoting benefits, you should have these in moderation (of course that's true of just about anything):

— **Dairy.** Be wary of dairy! Studies have shown that milk has a lot of steroid hormones and other compounds that may contribute to clogged pores, inflammation, and—yep—acne! How? It's believed that milk stimulates excess oil production, leaving pores sticky and susceptible to bacteria buildup. Also, it may cause hyperkeratinization (which means that the cells that line the hair follicle don't detach very often), leading to breakouts.

If you choose to restrict your consumption of dairy, make sure that you're getting your daily dose of vitamin D and calcium. Think of Popeye: eat lots of spinach, and strengthen those bones and biceps with weight training and exercise.

— **Caffeine.** Keep in mind that many beverages (such as energy drinks) and even medications contain caffeine, although the source may be listed as guarana or kola nut. Coffee dehydrates the skin, so you should limit your intake to no more than two cups a day. Dr. Rahm does believe that one cup a day is good for you, as coffee has antioxidant benefits. Try drinking an eight-ounce glass of water with the juice of half a lemon squeezed in it before you have your cup of joe—this will help neutralize the coffee's acid and is better for your skin.

— **Alcohol.** You should limit your alcohol intake to one to two drinks per day. If you want to enjoy a drink, opt for red wine, which contains the protective anti-aging compound called resveratrol. However, please note that one serving of wine is just five ounces.

Your Skin-surance Policy

To take supplements, or not to take supplements? I get asked all the time why I believe in taking them. Well, the truth is that most of us, no matter how hard we try, just don't eat the variety and quality of foods we need to eat daily to obtain *all* of the vitamins, minerals, antioxidants, and other phytonutrients we need to ensure radiant skin. Why not? There are lots of reasons, including that we're busy, we've skipped a meal, we've had an extra cup of coffee, we're dehydrated, or we didn't have any fresh veggies in the fridge when we started to cook dinner. Again, if we're eating conventionally grown foods, we're getting those that have been depleted of some of their natural nutrient content. And our body is in a delicate balance. It needs approximately 52 vitamins and minerals for all of the complex processes to function efficiently.

So how do you choose the right supplement for you? Much of what I know about nutritional supplements I learned from Dr. David Rahm. One important thing I learned is that, just like with professional skin-care products, there is a difference in quality, and you get what you pay for.

If you're already taking supplements and they're working for you, that's great. If not, here are a few tips for buying nutritional supplements:

■ Look at the inactive or "other" ingredients list to make sure that there is nothing you're allergic to. The eight common allergens are milk, eggs, fish, crustacean shellfish, peanuts, tree nuts, wheat, and soy.

■ If you are pregnant, are diabetic or have any other serious or chronic illness, or are getting ready to have surgery, talk to your doctor about taking supplements.

■ Follow the directions on how much to take. More is not necessarily better.

■ Buying in bulk may save you money, but it's not always a good idea. Some nutrients like vitamin C lose their potency over time, especially after they've been opened and are exposed to oxygen. Although not required by the FDA (Food and Drug Administration), do pay attention to expiration dates if they're provided.

- Store your supplements in a cool, dark place to maintain their shelf life.

- Like medications, keep nutritional supplements out of the reach of children and pets.

The Skin Health Pyramid, Part II: The Supplement Edition

In the same way that topical ingredients fit in to the Skin Health Pyramid, vitamins and minerals do too. I've categorized specific nutrients based on what function they best serve, be it to protect, hydrate, feed, stimulate, or detox. However, many nutrients tend to play multiple roles and serve several levels of the pyramid. Antioxidants, for instance, are such workhorses that they can fall into the protect, feed, *and* stimulate levels. So just know that while I've put each one into the level it best serves, many are performing for you on several levels. (Note that I've also included the RDA— or recommended daily allowance—of each ingredient, as noted by the United States government, wherever possible.)

Let's look at each level in detail now:

LEVEL I: PROTECT

— *Carotenoids.* Carotenoids, or carotenes, are fat-soluble plant compounds, some of which convert into vitamin A. Since beta-carotene converts the most readily, it's most often used in nutritional supplements. Other carotenes such as lycopene, zeaxanthin, astaxanthin, and lutein don't convert into vitamin A, but they still have potent antioxidant and protective benefits.

— *Vitamin E* is an antioxidant superhero that boosts healing and tissue repair and enhances immunity. For example, a German study showed that taking vitamin A with vitamin E reduced skin damage from sunburn. Look for products that offer a combination of tocopherols and tocotrienols. The RDA is 15 international units (IU).

— *Green-tea extract.* Green tea contains protective compounds called polyphenols that have antioxidant activity. In experiments with human skin, green-tea polyphenols showed anti-inflammatory and anti-carcinogenic properties.

— **Copper** is needed by your skin for the cross-linking of collagen and elastin and also for the formation of melanin, your natural sun protector. The RDA is 900 micrograms (mcg).

— **Selenium** is an important antioxidant and anti-inflammatory that can help alleviate psoriasis. Researchers have also found that selenium deficiency is common in people with metastatic melanoma. The RDA is 55 mcg.

LEVEL 2: HYDRATE

— **Essential fatty acids (EFAs).** The body can't produce these types of acids on its own, so you have to make sure you get enough in your diet. EFAs perform a number of vital functions, but they're particularly important at the cellular level: because cell membranes hold water in, the stronger they are, the better your skin cells can hold moisture.

Two essential fatty acids—alpha-linolenic acid (an omega-3) and linoleic acid (an omega-6)—are very important for a healthy body. In addition to alpha-linolenic acid, the omega-3 family of essential fatty acids includes EPA (eicosapentaenoic acid) and DHA (docosahexaenoic acid). As omega-3 fats, both EPA and DHA promote the development of favorable prostaglandins—hormonelike compounds—that play a role in inflammation, among other things. Flaxseed oil is one of the world's richest sources of omega-3s, and certain types of fish and fish oil contain high levels of EPA and DHA.

For most adults, one to two capsules of flaxseed oil and one to two capsules of fish oil a day will provide you with what you need. (Note that supplements should be packaged in bottles that do not expose the oil to damaging light or it can go off.) The only caveat I have is to start slowly if you're prone to oily skin.

— **Hyaluronic acid.** As you already know, hyaluronic acid is one of the skin's most important components for hydration and moisture retention. A high level of it can be found in the dermis, where it maintains the water balance and supports collagen and elastin. As we age, our ability to produce sufficient levels of hyaluronic acid diminishes, and as a result, the skin becomes drier. This is why I recommend that you supplement your diet with it.

— **The B complex** of vitamins help your body convert food into fuel, which is burned to produce energy; they're also necessary for healthy skin, hair, and eyes. You need this entire large group of important vitamins, but these Bs are particularly relevant to your skin:

- B_2 (riboflavin). If you don't get enough B_2, you can get some types of dermatitis, cracked lips, and increased sensitivity to sunlight. Yet you're only likely to get these symptoms if you eat a diet based mainly on processed white grains. The RDA is 1.1 milligrams (mg) for women and 1.3 mg for men.

- B_3 (niacin) helps make sex- and stress-related hormones in your adrenal glands and other parts of the body, and it improves circulation, too. The RDA is 16 to 18 mg for adults. (Note that high doses of niacin can cause your skin to flush.)

- B_5 (pantothenic acid) helps with wound healing, as it seems to cause cells to multiply. One study also showed that large doses help with acne, but this is not a widely used remedy. There is no RDA; suggested intake would be 5 mg.

- B_6 (pyridoxine). A deficiency of this vitamin can cause dermatitis-like symptoms, although it's rare. The RDA is 1.3 mg.

- B_7 (biotin) helps in the production of skin, nail, and hair cells. The RDA is 30 mcg.

- B_9 (folate) is particularly important for making and maintaining new cells, including skin cells. Studies have found that people with psoriasis (which is caused by cells that turn over too fast) often have a mild deficiency in folic acid. The RDA is 400 mcg.

- B_{12} (cobalamin) is critical for maintaining healthy red blood and nerve cells, and vegetarians and vegans sometimes don't get enough. The RDA is 2.4 mcg.

— **Vitamin D** is one of the vitamins that your body can manufacture as long as your skin is exposed to sunshine for 10 to 15 minutes, three times a week. A study at the University of California, San Diego School of Medicine seems to show that taking vitamin D boosts production of a protective chemical normally found in the skin, and it may help prevent skin infections suffered by people who have atopic dermatitis. The RDA for adults is 200 IU. However, that number goes up as we age: the RDA for men and women aged 50 to 70 is 400 IU, and then it's 600 IU for individuals over the age of 70.

— *Calcium* is a major player when it comes to skin health. The National Cancer Research Institute in the U.K. says that low amounts of calcium in our skin can make us more likely to experience premature aging and have a bigger risk for skin cancer. We also know that one symptom of low calcium may be eczema: scientists believe that this mineral regulates skin's cell growth and possibly its production of antioxidants. The RDA is 1,000 mg for adults; but men and women over the age of 50 should take 1,200 mg to maintain strong bones.

LEVEL 4: STIMULATE

— *Vitamin A* is like your skin's "maintenance man" in that it helps keep it operating properly. This vitamin repairs and reinforces the mucous membranes and tissues that protect against bacteria and viruses from entering your body. It keeps your skin from becoming dry, flaky, and wrinkled, and also helps prevent acne. As if that's not enough, vitamin A is an important antioxidant that purges your body of free radicals. The RDA is 700 mcg for women and 900 mcg for men.

— *Vitamin C* is vitally important to our bodies in general and our skin in particular. It's instrumental in forming amino acids and collagen, helps heal wounds, and is a well-known antioxidant that finds and fights free radicals. On top of that, vitamin C protects against infection and boosts our immune system. The RDA is 75 mg for women and 90 mg for men.

— *Magnesium* is required for a healthy immune system, among other things. It assists in the manufacturing of proteins and also offsets the effects of stress hormones. The RDA is 420 mg for men and 320 mg for women.

— *Zinc*, like vitamin C, helps cells regenerate collagen; it also helps with wound healing. The RDA is 11 mg for men and 9 mg for women—and if you're a vegetarian, you may need to take this mineral as a supplement. (Note that zinc competes with copper for absorption, so a high intake may create a copper deficiency.)

— **Alpha-lipoic acid.** This powerful antioxidant is hundreds of times more potent than either vitamin C or vitamin E. And like those vitamins, it helps neutralize skin-cell damage caused by free radicals. It's versatile in that it works in both fat- and water-soluble environments. Alpha-lipoic acid also regenerates other antioxidants.

— **Grapeseed extract** is a powerful antioxidant that strengthens collagen.

— **Ginkgo-biloba extract** is also a powerful antioxidant that is known for increasing circulation and has anti-aging properties.

— **Pycnogenol.** This antioxidant is extracted from the bark of the French maritime pine tree. In a 2004 study, researchers found that it selectively binds to collagen and elastin and protects them from degradation.

LEVEL 5: DETOX

— **Probiotics.** Whether they come in supplement, dairy, or nondairy form, probiotics help repopulate the gastrointestinal tract with the beneficial bacteria that are killed along with the bad bacteria when you take antibiotics. I generally recommend a limited dairy intake, but yogurt is a great source of this beneficial bacteria. Keep in mind, however, that it's best to choose a high-quality, preferably organic yogurt. As for probiotic supplements, excellent brands include Bio-K+ C1285 and Bifa-15, both of which can be found in health-food stores.

— **Botanicals.** Burdock, Oregon grape, dandelion, yellow dock, and milk thistle are often used in teas or supplements to help detoxify the blood and skin. Several studies have shown that low stomach acid is a common finding in patients with acne; therefore, the traditional use of bitter herbs, which act by stimulating digestive function or improving liver function, may be helpful.

A lifestyle and diet regimen, combined with the right treatment and product applications, is essential for anyone who is looking to dramatically change their skin, no matter what their skin type. And now it's time to find out what *your* skin type is . . . just turn the page.

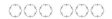

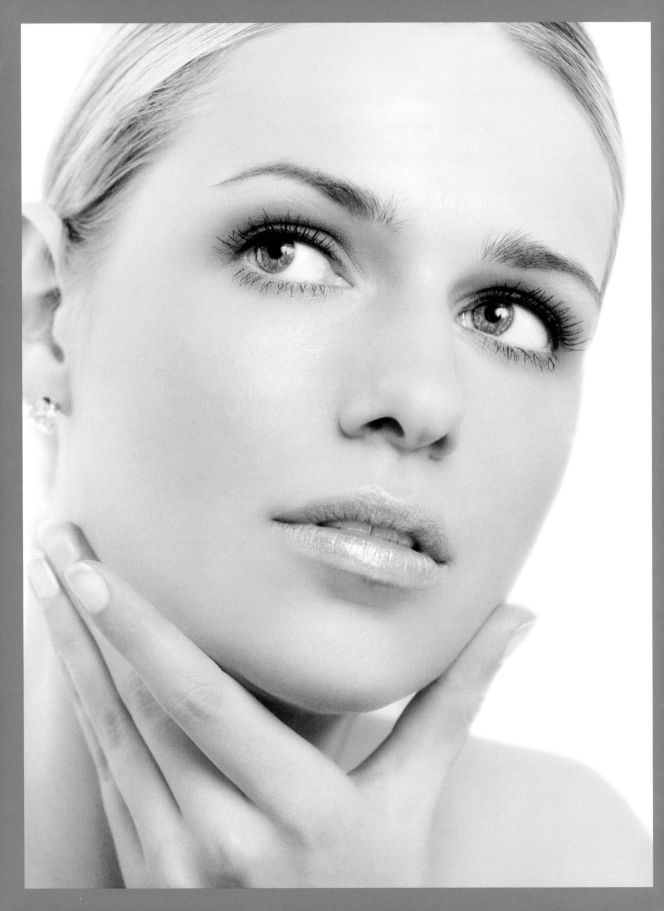

CHAPTER 5

What's Your Puzzle?

Are you ever puzzled by your skin—what's going on, why it's doing what it's doing, and how to fix it? If so, you'll understand why the first thing I do when a client walks into my clinic is ask a series of questions. I almost always say, "You're a puzzle. Let's figure you out." I want to get to know her skin and understand her concerns, issues, and goals.

I frequently tell my clients that our skin isn't always one way, all the time; rather, it has different "ecosystems." To illustrate what I mean, think about Maui. This small island has several distinct ecosystems all characterized by different weather patterns: it's cool and dry in the upper elevations; there are warm to hot interior areas; the windward areas are wet; there are even wetter low areas below the mountains; and there's the coastal, salt-spray zone.

Similarly, the face can be just as varied. While a lucky few of us have very balanced and temperate "climate conditions" on our faces, most of us don't. It can be calm and clear on the forehead, dry and patchy on the cheeks, and broken out on the chin.

So that's why it's crucial that I take a complete inventory of a new client's skin. I don't just look at her outside—I want to know what's going on inside as well. I want to know if she has allergies, sensitivities, or is on medications; if she's stressed-out, eats well, or exercises. I also want to know about her skin's history and how she personally feels about its present state. What does she love and appreciate about her complexion, and what would she like to change? As you can tell, I ask a lot of questions.

You should do the same. Get to know your own skin, both inside and out. The more connected you are to what's going on and how you feel, the better you can care for your skin puzzle now and throughout the years. Together, we're going to figure out your puzzle, and then we'll treat your skin according to whatever weather system has blown in. My goal for your skin is a balanced and beautiful ecosystem.

Connecting with Your Skin and Its Concerns

What follows will help you better connect with your skin. Please put a check mark next to any of these that you may have:

____ Fine lines and wrinkles

____ Facial folds around your mouth and/or nose

____ Rough skin texture

____ Enlarged pores

____ Tired-looking skin

____ Dry skin

____ Sagging skin

____ Uneven skin tone

____ Facial redness/rosacea

____ Brown spots/hyperpigmentation

____ Dark circles under your eyes

____ Thin lips

____ Acne

____ Acne scarring

____ Blackheads

____ Facial veins

____ Unwanted hair

____ Neck laxity

____ Allergies

____ Eczema

____ Psoriasis

Next, answer the following questions on a scale from 1 to 5 by circling the appropriate number:

When I look at my face in the mirror, I believe that I look younger, the same, or older than my true age:

Younger Than		True Age		Older Than
1	2	3	4	5

When looking in the mirror, I am concerned, somewhat concerned, or very concerned about the appearance of my wrinkles and/or skin laxity:

Not Concerned		Somewhat Concerned		Very Concerned
1	2	3	4	5

I eat a healthy diet—low in sugar, high in vegetables, organic whenever possible—and take necessary supplements:

Always		Sometimes		Never
1	2	3	4	5

I practice stress-reducing activities such as yoga, meditation, walking, gardening, massage, and socializing:

Always		Sometimes		Never
1	2	3	4	5

I exercise at least three times a week:

Always		Sometimes		Never
1	2	3	4	5

Now that we've taken inventory of your skin and lifestyle, you should have a better understanding of the current state of your complexion and your skin goals. This should help you identify your skin type from the charts that follow.

What's Your Skin Type?

It's important that you understand there's an infinite number of skin types and combinations. I know because I see so many combinations and unique cases walk through my clinic doors every day. For example, I see a lot of clients who have one type of skin on their forehead (dry), another type on their cheeks (rosacea), and another on their jawline (acne). There are also those clients whose skin actually changes on a regular basis: sunny one day, stormy the next. They could be a combination of three skin types over the course of a few months, depending on how hormonal they are and how their skin fluctuates. For this book, I've chosen to discuss the most common types I see, the ones I encounter all over the globe.

The charts in this chapter identify 13 common skin types: the left side outlines the characteristics of each, while the right side offers my goals for each type. Read through them, and identify your own—finding your skin type and understanding what's listed in the next few pages will be a great jumping-off point for you as we move into the next part of the book.

SKIN TYPE: NORMAL

CHARACTERISTICS	GOALS
■ Healthy and balanced, smooth to the touch	■ Maintain the health and balance of the skin
■ Soft and luminous	■ Keep skin texture firm and healthy
■ Smaller pores, free of congestion	■ Prevent fine lines and wrinkles from forming
■ Not characterized by spots or sun damage	
■ Even tone and texture; firm and elastic	
■ Not sensitive to many products or ingredients	

SKIN TYPE: DRY

CHARACTERISTICS

- Lacks natural oil and hydration
- Characterized by fine lines and general dullness
- Can be flaky in spots or have dry patches
- Pores tend to be small
- Lips are often chapped, and darker skin types can appear ashy

GOALS

- Improve hydration levels and luminosity
- Get skin glowing
- Reduce lines associated with dehydration
- Plump up skin cells and reduce irritation associated with dryness

SKIN TYPE: SENSITIVE

CHARACTERISTICS

- Prone to redness and sensitivity
- Highly reactive to products and ingredients
- May break out from topical treatments or even certain foods
- Skin can sometimes be thin and very dry

GOALS

- Identify sensitivities and avoid products, ingredients, and foods that contribute to this
- Reduce inflammation
- Strengthen the skin's immune system
- Balance and even skin tone
- Reduce blotchiness or redness

SKIN TYPE: OILY

CHARACTERISTICS

- Shiny and greasy to the touch, especially in the T-zone: forehead, nose, and chin
- Enlarged pores, orange-peel-like texture
- Frequently congested with blackheads; prone to breakouts

GOALS

- Control sebum production
- Eliminate excess shine and promote a healthy glow
- Reduce pore size and clear skin of blackheads

SKIN TYPE: COMBINATION

CHARACTERISTICS	GOALS
■ Can be oily and congested in the T-zone	■ Balance the skin and keep it even in tone
■ Other areas may be drier, with scaly patches	■ Control areas prone to oiliness and moisturize areas that are dry
■ Surface dryness can also occur, with oiliness underneath	■ Keep skin well exfoliated so that it appears even and tight
■ Breakouts can appear in clusters	

SKIN TYPE: ACNE

CHARACTERISTICS	GOALS
■ Breaks out often	■ Create a healthy and smooth complexion
■ Has blemishes and eruptions, both on the surface of the skin and underneath	■ Clear up breakouts and prevent future ones
■ Acne can be in the form of superficial whiteheads, blackheads, and generalized congestion; or in the form of cysts that occur under the surface of the skin	■ Eliminate sensitivities, detox the skin, and keep pores clean and clear
■ May have discoloration due to past breakouts	■ Balance oil production and improve texture
	■ Get rid of surface dryness and inflammation
	■ Restore skin to a smooth complexion, free of eruptions
	■ Lighten pigmentation caused by past breakouts

SKIN TYPE: MATURE

CHARACTERISTICS	GOALS
■ Generally associated with a thinning of the skin	■ Restore a youthful radiance to the complexion
■ Fine lines around the eyes and lips, with deeper expression lines forming around the mouth and forehead	■ Reduce lines and add volume to the skin
■ Undereye area has bags and darker circles	■ Increase the collagen and elastin levels within the dermis
■ Often dry	■ Soften lip lines, folds, and crow's-feet
	■ Tighten the skin and brighten the undereye area

SKIN TYPE: MATURE AND ACNE

CHARACTERISTICS	GOALS
■ Maturing skin, with loss of elasticity and skin tone	■ Reduce pore size, fine lines, and wrinkles, and clear up breakouts
■ Fine lines and deeper lines, depending on age	■ Restore a healthy glow to the skin and improve overall texture
■ Blemishes frequently occur in the "U-zone" around jawline and on cheeks	■ Keep breakouts under control, while preventing new lines from forming
■ Adult acne is often cystic, with raised bumps under the skin's surface and congested, enlarged pores	■ Work to get skin as balanced as possible
	■ Hydrate and moisturize, without causing breakouts

SKIN TYPE: HYPERPIGMENTED

CHARACTERISTICS	GOALS
■ Spots and freckling darker than the natural skin color, caused by sun exposure	■ Lighten pigmentation and sun spots
■ Spots can be very light in color or darker pigmented	■ Create an even skin tone and color
	■ Prevent future spots from forming

SKIN TYPE: HYPERPIGMENTED/MELASMA

CHARACTERISTICS	GOALS
■ Associated with hormonal fluctuation and sometimes referred to as a "pregnancy mask"	■ Lighten masking and restore the skin's natural, even pigmentation
■ Skin has darker, brownish pigment in certain areas, and is most often blotchy and symmetrical	■ Melasma is stubborn, so the goal is also to keep it from appearing again

SKIN TYPE: SCARRED

CHARACTERISTICS

- Often a result of past acne, skin can be marked by brown or red spots
- Some scarring creates divots or pits in the skin, where there is uneven texture and loss of collagen

GOALS

- Stimulate collagen and elastin
- Flatten out scarring
- Improve overall texture
- Brighten the overall complexion
- Even out uneven tone caused by scarring

SKIN TYPE: ROSACEA

CHARACTERISTICS

- Abnormal redness on the cheeks and nose are most common
- Small blood vessels are visible on the face and can make a weblike pattern
- In more severe cases, tiny, acne-like raised bumps can form

GOALS

- Soften generalized redness
- Rid the skin of rosacea, bumps, and broken capillaries
- Create a smoother, more refined texture
- Reduce the thickened state of the skin
- Even skin color and tone

SKIN TYPE: ECZEMA

CHARACTERISTICS

- Dry, rough patches on the skin; persistent flakiness
- Often itchy, uncomfortable, and irritated; flare-ups are common

GOALS

- Get eczema into remission
- Achieve healthy, balanced skin; free of dry, thickened patches
- Improve and even out texture
- Strengthen the immunity of skin

So now it's time to get down to the nitty-gritty—and my favorite part—all of those treatments, products, and ingredients that really work for beautiful skin. I want you to know what's available and effective; and to be able to determine what's best for you based on your goals, your budget, your lifestyle, and your skin type.

The next part of this book will simplify things for you, in that it will serve as a guide on your journey toward complexion perfection.

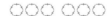

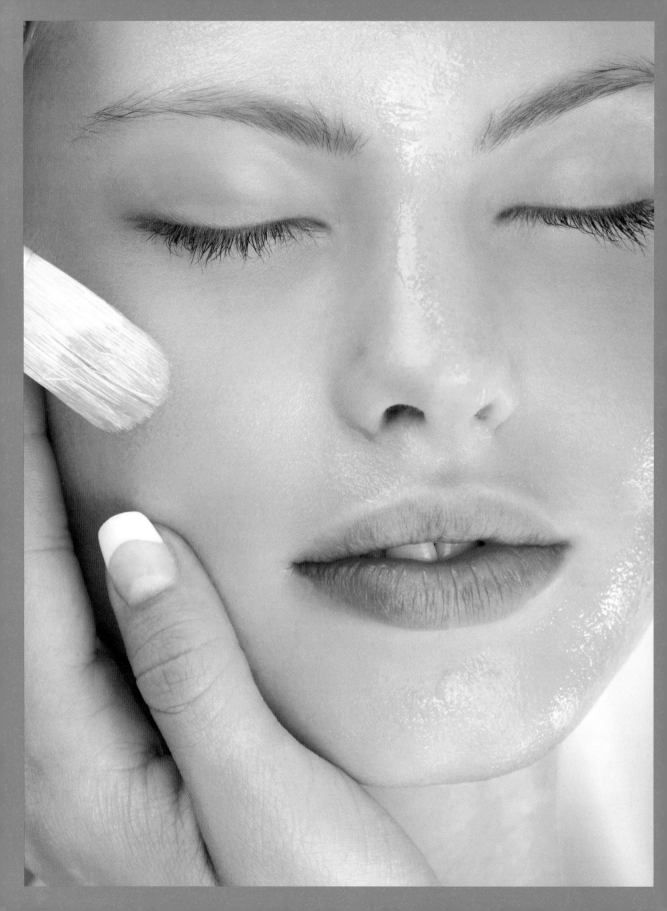

PART II

Complexion Correction!

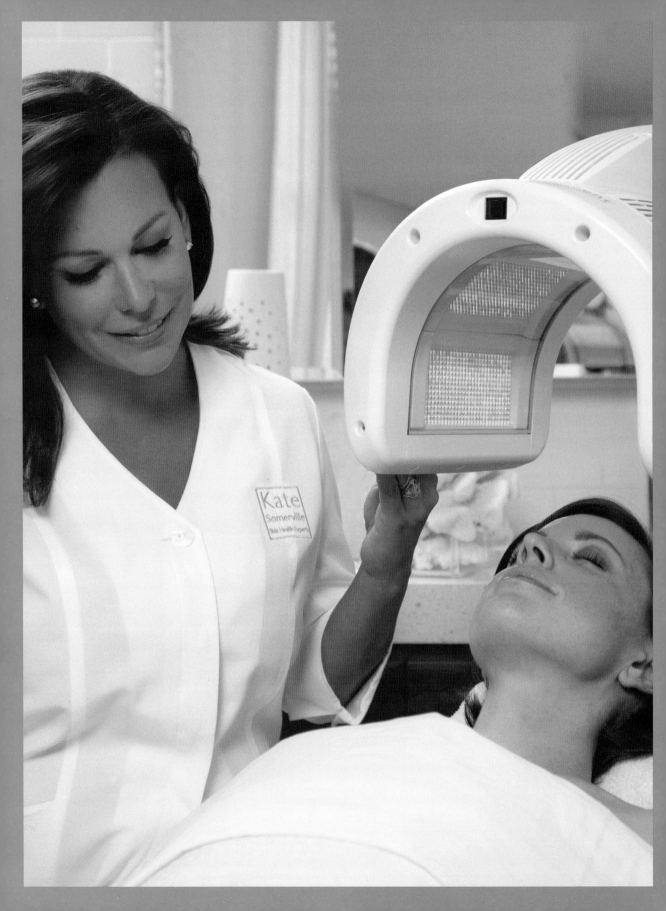

CHAPTER 6

Treatments That Transform

It's an exciting time in skin care, and I feel so lucky to be a part of this age of discovery. We have the ability to deliver healthy, radiant, ageless skin without taking the extreme risks associated with strategies of the past. However, this can also be a confusing time in that you can't turn on the television, flip through a magazine, or surf the Internet without being bombarded by information on products or services that promise amazing results.

Many are expensive, have hard-to-pronounce ingredients, and involve treatments that sound strange and scary. Incredible solutions do exist that deliver real results, but how are you to know what is safe, effective, and right for you?

I understand just how confusing it is. I am presented with virtually every treatment, product, ingredient, and packaging innovation on the market and have to sift through it all to figure out what's safe and effective. For me, that's always been the bottom line: *What works? What changes skin?* And I've done my research. I've spent my entire professional career getting to the bottom of skin issues and solving them. Today when I come up against a really difficult acne or pigmentation case, or if someone just isn't responding to my treatment program, I don't give up. I introduce a new treatment strategy or adjust the product regimen until I see results.

Years ago, I didn't have the safe tools I needed to solve severe cystic acne, but today, thanks to technology, I can. And that makes me feel so good. Clients with virtually every skin type and condition have crossed the threshold of my clinic, and my technicians and I work to either help them *achieve* healthy skin or *keep* it healthy. I've had the pleasure of getting to the bottom of thousands of challenging cases over the years. As a woman with her own issues, I've also tried many things myself, so not only do I have a professional opinion, but I've got a personal one, too.

This chapter details the treatments I believe are safe and deliver results. I want you to be educated and informed so that you can be in charge of your own transformation. I'm including treatments that can be performed by an esthetician, such as facials and LED treatments, and those that need to be done by a registered nurse or doctor, such as laser treatments and injectables.

Technology can be expensive. We all know that when a new cell phone or computer comes on the market, it's usually pricey and then gets more affordable after a few years. The same can be true of skin care. Some established, effective services are very reasonable, while others—usually the cutting-edge ones—come with a higher price tag. I think the most important thing is to understand your skin, your budget, and your goals. There are affordable solutions out there, but it's important to do your research and realize that the cheapest option is not necessarily the best one.

I'm always surprised by people who spend a lot of money on a designer handbag or a high-tech gadget and yet feel uncomfortable spending money on their skin. You wear your face every day, and this is what meets the world. So when considering your spending choices, I strongly believe your skin is a worthwhile investment, just like your monthly haircut and/or color services.

Who Can You Trust?

When you do decide to make that investment in yourself, I want you to walk into that doctor's office or skin-care clinic and be educated and knowledgeable about the services and products that exist. Also, I want you to understand that not all services or treatments are suitable for everyone. If you have a bad reaction to something you've been given by a dermatologist or esthetician, you'll probably think, *Oh, I can't ever go back to that place.* The truth is, that person can't possibly know everything about your skin right away; he or she goes through a process of learning about you and how your skin reacts and responds. One of the most important pieces of advice I can give you is: work with your skin-care professional. It should be a partnership—if it doesn't feel that way, then I absolutely recommend seeking someone else.

Selecting your professional is very, very important, so do some homework. Get to know the person who will be taking care of you and your skin issues. Ask for references from recent clients, or go to someone recommended by a friend who's happy with her results and the entire experience. You can also ask to see before-and-after pictures, which can be helpful and revealing. But be sure these are pictures of the practitioner's work, not those supplied by the manufacturer of the treatment.

Always ask this question: "How long have you been doing this particular treatment?" That's much more relevant than, "How long have you been in business?" All of us in the industry have a learning curve with a new system or treatment or injectable. When someone is learning, there is more risk. But believe it or not, I've encountered doctors who have been practicing for decades who actually have too much confidence! They can be "cowboys" who will grab a laser and start firing away with it before they really know what they're doing.

Technology is moving at a record pace, and the cosmetics industry is big business. Not all practitioners are qualified, even if they say they are. Doctors of all sorts are opening up their clinics to cosmetic procedures—and be especially aware of those who advertise that they're the first to be using a new treatment that has just been FDA approved. It's always best to select a professional who is trained and experienced. When I hire a new nurse, for instance, she doesn't work on clients for at least three months. Extensive training is one of the cornerstones of my clinic, and it should be important to you when you're selecting your doctor's office or skin clinic.

Over the years, I've learned something else. Treatments and technologies are promoted by established companies, and many of us assume that the company has done the research and has treatment protocol perfectly figured out. *If it's out there,*

A Hairy Story

A few years ago, a renowned actor came to me with major pigmentation and scarring on his back and shoulders. It turns out that he'd gone to a well-known dermatologist's office for laser hair removal right after having spent some time in the sun. You see, laser hair removal works this way: the laser is attracted to the dark pigment in the hair at the follicle. If you're darker skinned (or have a tan like he did) and the technician isn't using caution, the laser can be attracted to the skin's natural pigment or to the tan. This can cause a terrible-looking checkerboard pattern on the skin . . . and unfortunately, that's what happened.

The worst part of it was that he had to film a major motion picture three weeks later and had to film scenes with his shirt off! When he came to us in search of a solution, we did a series of peels on his back to get rid of the discoloration and even out the pigment. But we didn't have enough time to totally reverse the damage, so we had to send a self-tanning specialist to the set for on-the-spot camouflage work.

My husband and I went to see his movie, and at the end of the day, this actor looked great on-screen. You may have seen him yourself, and of course you would have had no idea what he went through to look that way.

we think, *it must be safe*. But that's not always the case. Although the FDA does a really good job, their approval doesn't always mean that the product or technology is perfect. However, the best practitioners will always work with companies and brands that have a good track record with safety and efficacy.

What Works Where

Products and treatments are designed to be effective at different depths and on different layers of the skin. To get the healthiest, youngest-looking skin, you have to take care of it at every level.

Today, skin health and treatment are multidimensional. Once, face-lifts were the only way to turn back time, and they really only address one dimension of the skin: sagging. But as you now know, there are many layers and levels that need to be addressed: the epidermis, the dermis, the subcutaneous fatty tissue, the muscle, and all the way down to the bone. And every level ages in its own unique way. We lose elasticity, which causes sagging; we lose fat and collagen, which causes the loss of firmness and volume; and we lose plumpness in the dermis because hyaluronic acid is depleting and production of it is slowing. All of this leads to lines and dullness. Skin begins to thin, the surface begins to show spots, pores stretch, and we lose our youthful glow. The facial muscles fall with age and gravity, and our bones even shrink as we age. So understand that in order to age beautifully, you have to protect and preserve *every* dimension of your skin, from the top layer down to the bone.

(A quick note before we discuss treatment: if you are pregnant or have certain allergies or health conditions, please check with your health-care provider before trying anything in this chapter.)

Let's take another look at that diagram of the skin you saw in Chapter I. Because we age on different levels, this diagram illustrates what treatments work and where:

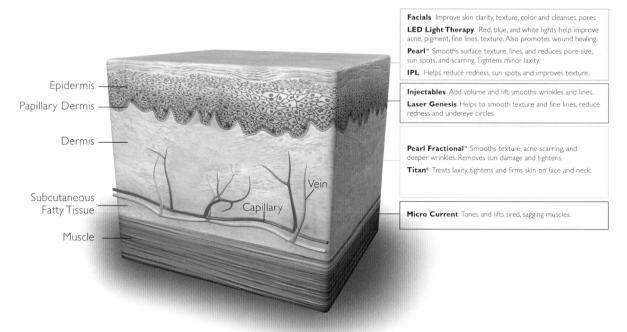

Facials Improve skin clarity, texture, color and cleanses pores
LED Light Therapy Red, blue, and white lights help improve acne, pigment, fine lines, texture. Also promotes wound healing.
Pearl™ Smooths surface texture, lines, and reduces pore size, sun spots, and scarring. Tightens minor laxity.
IPL Helps reduce redness, sun spots, and improves texture.

Injectables Add volume and lift, smooths wrinkles and lines.
Laser Genesis Helps to smooth texture and fine lines, reduce redness and undereye circles.

Pearl Fractional™ Smooths texture, acne scarring, and deeper wrinkles. Removes sun damage and tightens.
Titan® Treats laxity, tightens and firms skin on face and neck.

Micro Current Tones and lifts tired, sagging muscles.

Epidermis
Papillary Dermis
Dermis
Subcutaneous Fatty Tissue
Muscle
Vein
Capillary

The rest of the chapter will discuss each of the skin treatments mentioned in the diagram—and many more—in detail.

Facials and Related Services

Facials, whether you have them done by a professional or do them at home, are an important component of healthy skin. These treatments address the top layers of the skin, mostly the epidermis.

One of the most popular facials at my clinic is called the DermalQuench Oxygen Therapy. The esthetician begins by exfoliating the skin with enzymes and gentle acids. She then uses an airbrush applicator to push a serum that's formulated with vitamins and hyaluronic acid into the skin cells. She finishes with the application of a moisturizer that's packed with peptides, rich emollients, and ingredients to further lock in hydration. This treatment is particularly beloved by celebrities who are about to hit red-carpet events because it ups the hydration level in their skin, keeping it supple, hydrated, smooth, and dewy. All facials, however, will greatly improve the health and appearance of your skin, so be sure to get them regularly. And if it's outside of your budget, do them yourself! In Chapter 8, I'll tell you how to do just that.

REGULAR FACIALS

— *What it is:* A professional facial usually involves a thorough cleaning and exfoliation; steam to open your pores; extractions (the removal of blackheads, whiteheads, and pimples) if necessary; a moisturizing or tightening mask, depending on your needs; perhaps a facial massage; and, finally, the application of serums and moisturizers. I think that regular facials are crucial because they're a way for you and your skin-care professional to keep tabs on changes in your skin health.

— *Who it's for:* Everyone. Facials should be customized to your skin type, and the products used in them should work specifically on your unique needs and goals.

— *What to expect:* Skin should look brighter, clearer, healthier, and balanced.

— *Know this:* You can give yourself a simplified facial at home (see Chapter 8 for details).

— *Estimated cost:* Anywhere from $85 to $200 for a professional service.

DERMAPLANING

— *What it is:* A professional treatment that involves manual exfoliation. It's a gentle scraping of the skin's surface with a blade.

— *Who it's for:* Dry skin types or those with surface dryness and oiliness underneath. It also helps improve pigmentation or acne scarring. And it's great for getting rid of "peach fuzz" on the face.

— *What to expect:* The treatment can be combined with a facial and improves the results of IPL (you'll learn more about this later) when performed immediately before, and then one week after, treatment. It's simple, requires no downtime, and will leave skin very smooth and soft.

— *Know this:* Although this is an incredibly safe procedure, make sure that your practitioner is experienced in dermaplaning. After all, he or she will be working with a really sharp blade!

— *Estimated cost:* $50 to $75.

ULTRASOUND TREATMENTS

— *What it is:* A handheld device used to deliver sound waves into the top layers of the skin to improve cellular metabolism and skin tone, texture, and clarity. It can usually be incorporated in, or added to, a regular facial.

— *Who it's for:* Most skin types will benefit. Ultrasound treatments have been found to be highly effective in wound healing because they stimulate fibroblasts to produce collagen. They detoxify the skin and are therefore good for acne. Also, when used in combination with lightening agents, ultrasound increases product penetration and can improve and brighten pigmentation over time.

— *What to expect:* You will experience improved skin tone, smoothness, and texture. You may also notice an increase in the hydration levels of your skin. It is comfortable and may feel a little tingly.

— *Know this:* Ultrasound wavelengths at 3 MHZ is the correct level of energy for the skin and is safe.

— *Estimated cost:* $75 to $200.

MICROCURRENT

— *What it is:* Very small electrical impulses that mimic those naturally occurring in the body. They trigger chemical reactions at the cellular level to encourage the production of collagen and elastin. Additionally, microcurrent helps bring oxygen to the skin cell by enhancing circulation. A popular treatment at my clinic, it also works to reeducate muscles and lift them back into shape—think of it as a gym for the skin. When done well, microcurrent can sculpt and contour the facial muscles for a firm, plump, and youthful result.

— *Who it's for:* This treatment is great to start in your early 30s, when you begin to see those cheeks deflate. It's great before a big event, as the results are immediate. Also, the effects of regular microcurrent treatments are cumulative and will add up to incredibly toned and elastic skin.

— *What to expect:* Usually the facialist will use two sets of prongs to sculpt your face, gently coaxing the muscles into a more lifted position. You may feel a slight tingle, or even a sharper one in sensitive areas. We like to do one side of the face, and then show the client the lifted brow, cheek, and jawline before beginning the other side.

— *Know this:* If you have any metal fillings, you may notice the slight taste of metal in your mouth. However, if the tingle is incredibly intense, this means that the energy is too high and should be lowered. This is one treatment where pain does not equal gain. You want the microcurrent to mimic the subtlety of the body's own electricity, so you shouldn't be jumping out of the chair!

— *Estimated cost:* $150 to $350 per treatment.

Clinical/Medical Skin Treatments

The treatments I discuss in the next several pages are those that, in most states, must be performed by a medical professional or under the guidance of a medical director. There are many options out there, so I've narrowed it down to the ones that we perform at my clinic or that I've seen used safely, successfully, and with great results. In fact, I've had many of these treatments myself, and so have members of my staff.

At my clinic, we often combine treatments and products for custom-designed programs, so we can achieve the best results. However, the treatments that follow can be found in dermatologists' offices and skin-care clinics across the nation. Some you may have heard of, while I'm sure others will be new to you.

Often, when clients walk in my door, they're really confused about fillers and what they can do. So let's set things straight. Fillers address the loss of volume and fullness as we age, especially in the dermal and fat layers. The skin gradually loses hydration and its fat cushion, but fillers can reintroduce natural-looking volume and plumpness associated with youthful skin. These can really change someone's face, and do so instantly.

Fillers can be applied under the eyes wherever there are depressions, circles, and pockets. They can also be used to add fullness to the lips and fill in the surrounding lines. They can add volume to the cheeks and are incredibly effective in softening smile lines.

When applied strategically, fillers look very natural and can take years off of the face by lifting and plumping. However, they are injected, and their application is an art form—things can go badly if you go to someone who isn't skilled. I think we've all seen this: overplumped lips, uneven distribution, or even worse.

I like to use fillers very subtly, and work with many that are on the market. Some are firm, while others are softer, depending on the consistency of the substance. I have found that some work best in specific areas. At my clinic, we sometimes use five different fillers for different parts of the face. Let's say that someone has a beautiful bottom lip, but a very thin top lip. We'll even that out and create more balance—for the lip line, we'll use Restylane®, and then in the soft part of the lip, we'll use Juvéderm®.

Injectables are moldable, and we have about 24 hours to push the substance around or press and pinch it into shape. Our nurses do this for our clients, and we teach our clients how to do it as well. Generally, clients will come in twice for fillers. They usually get some swelling at first, so we like to see them after that has subsided and do some touch-up work. We also recommend taking arnica, a homeopathic anti-inflammatory, and bromelain, a natural enzyme that helps with bruising. (Or you can eat pineapple, which is naturally high in bromelain!) Bruising is generally unavoidable, but the touch of the technician is very important. If he or she rushes and is hardhanded, there's more chance for increased bruising.

Another great thing is that if you don't like what you see, or don't like the substance you've had injected, most fillers have an antidote that will help dissolve them. There are also lasers that can break down the substance, so you're not stuck with a look you're unhappy with. In any event, the results are not permanent, and most injectables dissolve naturally, generally lasting from three months to a year.

Here's some detailed information about the three most popular types of injectable fillers:

1. Hyaluronic-Acid Fillers

— *What it is:* Hyaluronic acid is a natural substance found in the human body that cushions and lubricates joints, eyes, and heart valves; it also plumps and hydrates skin. In gel form, it becomes my favorite filler, which is injected into wrinkles and folds. The brands we use are Juvéderm, Restylane, and Perlane®, all of which are FDA approved.

— *Who it's for:* Those who want to hydrate and add volume to the skin. These types of fillers smooth deep lines like those from your nose to your lips (nasolabial folds) and at the corners of your mouth (marionette lines), fill in the hollows under the eyes, and can sculpt lips.

— *What to expect:* You'll see results immediately (or in some cases, within a couple of days), and they can last anywhere from 6 to 12 months.

— *Know this:* Minimally invasive, these injections have no downtime. You might get some minor swelling that goes down in a couple of days. I like to use Juvéderm in the lips and Restylane or Perlane under the eyes. Also, because these products create a cushion, they help prevent future wrinkles from forming.

— *Estimated cost:* $300 to $600 per syringe, based on size.

2. Radiesse®

— *What it is:* Radiesse is a dermal filler made from synthetic calcium-based microspheres suspended in a water-based gel. It's injected into deep folds and any sunken areas where you've lost underlying fat. It also stimulates your body's own collagen production. Radiesse is FDA approved.

— *Who it's for:* Those who want to fill, smooth, and contour their skin for a rejuvenated look. Radiesse is best used in the cheekbone area or anywhere you want to contour.

— *What to expect:* You can expect to see results right away, and they can last a year or longer.

— *Know this:* Minimally invasive, this treatment can have "social" downtime. This means that you can go about your daily business but won't want to schedule any special events, since you might experience some short-term redness, bruising, or swelling. The microspheres can be detected in x-rays and CT scans, so you should inform your doctor if you need to undergo these procedures. Because Radiesse does last longer than most fillers, you should be confident with the technician you're choosing and very clear about the look you want to achieve. I don't recommend this in the eye or lip area.

— *Estimated cost:* Around $800 per syringe.

3. Collagen Fillers

— *What they are:* Made from purified human-based collagen, these fillers are injected into the collagen layer of your dermis. **Please note:** These products have been discontinued; as of this writing, they were still on the market, but they may not be available by the time you read this book.

BOTOX® COSMETIC

There is some confusion about fillers and Botox. Fillers do just that: fill in hollows and creases. Botox is completely different: it slows muscle contraction to prevent lines from forming. Ideally, the two can be used together. In my clinic, we like to use Botox first to relax clients' muscles and then use fillers; that way, their muscles won't displace the filler. Plus, they might need less filler after Botox.

Botox can be abused if it's administered in the wrong place or too much is used. Yes, we've all seen that "alien forehead"—frozen, flat, and expressionless. As with fillers, its application is also an art form. And the technician needs to take the whole face into account; if she doesn't, what happens is that she'll stop some expression lines, but they'll show up somewhere else. For example, if she totally freezes forehead frown lines, the client can end up with what I call "bunny nose": horizontal creases at the bridge of the nose between the eyes.

Just tiny dots of well-placed Botox around your face can even things up and give you a natural, smooth look while leaving you with the ability to form expressions. Think about it: I work on a lot of actors, and they do not want to be expressionless!

— *What it is:* Botox is a sterile, purified version of the toxin botulism. Small amounts are injected into your muscles to temporarily block nerve impulses that signal the muscles to contract. Minimally invasive, it's the most popular and fastest-growing cosmetic procedure. The FDA approves Botox for cosmetic use in people age 18 to 65.

— *Who it's for:* People in their 20s who want to prevent creases caused by expression lines, and those in their 30s and beyond who want to erase them. Most often Botox is used on frown lines, laugh lines, and the fine lines above the lip. When applied correctly, it can also lift the brows and upper eyelids. It is frequently used in conjunction with injectable fillers.

— *What to expect:* You'll see some results in just a few days, but it will take a couple of weeks for the muscles to relax. Those results will last approximately three to four months.

— *Know this:* The procedure only takes a few minutes and there is no downtime. (Yet some people do have short-lived side effects such as a droopy eyelid, nausea, and mild redness and pain at the site of the injection.) You can even use a tiny bit above the lip to reduce a "gummy" smile.

— *Estimated cost:* $150 to $800.

LASERS

Since the 1980s, the laser has been a key technology in cosmetic procedures. Lasers can vary from being nonablative, which means no or very little (three to five days) downtime, to really ablative, where the recovery time can mean weeks or even months. Lasers in skin care have come a long way in recent years, and I personally believe in and use nonablative treatments. My busy clients simply can't afford to take the time off for anything longer.

As with injectables, there's a lot of confusion about lasers, and I understand why. There are so many out there, and they can treat a variety of skin conditions and concerns, from acne and pigmentation to refining pores, reducing wrinkles, and tightening skin. Some lasers hurt, some are mildly uncomfortable, and some are more or less pain free, as you'll see with the following four treatments. Note that these four are the ones that I either use or believe to be safe and effective.

1. Titan®

— *What it is:* Titan is a really simple procedure: a laser that heats the dermis, adding thickness to the skin. It stimulates your collagen to tighten sagging and reduce wrinkles and can be used on your face and neck—I call it the nonsurgical face-lift. Titan is the first light-based system approved by the FDA for the safe treatment of lax skin.

— *Who it's for:* People losing elasticity, who are seeing signs of "turkey neck," drooping jowls, and a downturned mouth. I've seen it take five to ten years off of a face. It can also be used for minor acne scarring and to reduce pitting, and it's suitable for all skin types.

— *What to expect:* Some people get good results with one treatment, while others need up to three. Although you'll often notice some immediate results, you'll see optimal benefits in three to six months as your collagen responds to the treatment.

— *Know this:* A few people get some redness and a little bit of swelling immediately after the procedure, but it only lasts an hour or so. I frequently recommend the Titan for my celeb clients because there is absolutely no downtime. It's so safe that we can do it the night before the Oscars and the Emmy Awards.

— *Estimated cost:* $1,200 to $2,500 per treatment.

2. Pearl®

— *What it is:* Pearl actually takes down a layer of skin by way of a laser for quick results. At the same time, it sends heat to deeper levels for longer-term benefits. This treatment is FDA approved for treating wrinkles.

— *Who it's for:* My team uses the Pearl on all ages because it reduces wrinkles, pore size, fine lines, uneven texture, sun damage, and pigmentation. And in my opinion, it's off the charts for acne scarring. However, the Pearl cannot be used on darker skin types.

— *What to expect:* For general tightening and brightening, one treatment will give you a very smooth texture (like a pearl!) in about seven days. If you have severe scarring, I recommend three treatments, and then you'll see longer-term improvement in texture and tone.

— *Know this:* The skin is cleansed and then numbed with a cream for about 30 to 45 minutes prior to the treatment. Each pulse of the Pearl feels like a hot rubber-band snap. In addition, the skin feels very warm immediately after the treatment, so over-the-counter pain medicine is suggested if all this is too uncomfortable. The treatment has about four to seven days of social downtime. You get red—it looks a bit like windburn—and then the skin gets very dry and begins to flake off. You also have to use an ointment on your face for a couple of days and completely avoid the sun.

— *Estimated cost:* $1,000 to $2,000 per treatment.

3. Pearl Fractional®

— *What it is:* This is a newer procedure that's a combination of the Pearl and Titan. The Pearl Fractional is a little more invasive than the regular Pearl treatment because it penetrates the dermis, vaporizes and removes damaged tissue, and stimulates new cell growth as the skin repairs itself.

— *Who it's for:* It's great for acne scarring, as well as deep lines, enlarged pores, pigmentation, and skin laxity.

— *What to expect:* Most people only need one treatment to see quite dramatic results.

— *Know this:* Downtime is seven to ten days.

— *Estimated cost:* Around $3,000 per treatment.

4. Laser Genesis®

— *What it is:* This is a noninvasive laser technology using near infrared light and heat to get down to the dermis to stimulate collagen production and healthy cell growth. I call it my "skin polisher," since it smooths out the surface layers, too. Laser Genesis is also great for gradually building volume and reducing redness, not to mention for textural issues such as "orange peel" skin and fine lines. This is one of my personal favorite treatments.

— *Who it's for:* Anyone with fine lines or texture issues such as large pores and scarring; it also reduces redness in dilated capillaries. It's fantastic for people with a ruddy complexion caused by deep rosacea. For acne, it helps clear up outbreaks and blemish-causing bacteria. It can be used on any skin type or color.

— *What to expect:* For optimal outcomes, most people need six to eight treatments. At first, results are subtle, but the accumulative, long-term effects can be quite dramatic.

— *Know this:* The procedure is totally painless and, in fact, can feel quite relaxing. At most you may get some mild redness immediately after treatment, but it fades within hours. There is no downtime.

— *Estimated cost:* $200 to $500 per treatment.

LIGHT THERAPIES

I. Omnilux™ LED Technology

— *What it is:* Omnilux is a combination of noninvasive blue, red, and white LED technology (also referred to as "light-emitting diode," "light treatment," or "phototherapy") that's used both for acne treatment and to combat aging. (In addition, the red and white lights are used in burn units and after surgery for those people who are slow to heal.) Note that in other clinics, the white LED is also referred to as the near infrared LED.

I started using LED technology about a year after I opened my clinic. Before that, I had about a 60 percent success rate in treating acne with topical products. But ever since I added in the LED treatments, I have a more than *90 percent* success rate in treating acne. It greatly changed the way I take care of the clients in my clinic.

— *Who it's for:*

■ Omnilux can *really* help teens with acne. I want parents to know that this is a far better option than internal drugs and even topical drugs for their kids. The blue and red LED eradicate the bacteria that cause the inflammation experienced during breakouts, reduce pore size, stabilize sebum production, and promote healthy cell growth. It's also good for anyone of any age with acne.

■ For the effects of aging, red and white lights stimulate collagen and elastin production to stimulate your skin's own ability to heal and rejuvenate. They soften lines and even skin tone over time.

— *What to expect:*

■ For acne, the treatment course is two treatments—one blue light, one red light—weekly for four weeks. More than one course may be necessary if you have severe cystic acne. You should see results within 12 weeks. I often combine light treatments with topical creams for extreme acne to enhance or speed up the results.

■ For anti-aging, red and white lights are prescribed as needed, often in conjunction with other treatments such as lasers, injectables, and serums. You'll see some immediate results, and your skin can continue to improve for up to six months. I recommend adding lights to your monthly facial for maintenance.

— *Know this:* Your eyes will be protected. The lights are positioned very close to your face and can make some people feel claustrophobic. The red light is particularly intense and it takes a few minutes for your eyes to adjust. The first time I tried it, I was like, "Whoa!" But this treatment is totally safe, although not recommended for people with immune deficiencies. At our clinic, we call these treatments our DermaLucent technologies.

Some dermatologists are using a combination of white light with topical chemotherapy to eradicate basal cell carcinomas and squamous cell carcinomas, rather than cutting them out.

— *Estimated cost:* $100 to $200 per treatment, but they're often sold in packages to reduce the price.

2. Intense Pulsed Light Therapy (IPL)

— *What it is:* IPL is a generic term, and you'll find the treatment under names like Photofacial and Solar Genesis. These systems are different from lasers in that they deliver many colors in each pulse of light instead of just one. It's a shortwave light that hits the skin, targeting discolored or damaged surface layers and delivering heat deeper in the dermis to stimulate healing. While this treatment can help a bit with surface lines, it won't tighten the skin.

— *Who it's for:* IPL is highly effective for fair-skinned people with hyperpigmentation, freckles, broken capillaries, sun damage, age spots, and surface rosacea (but not deep rosacea). It also reduces pore size and refines the overall texture and tone of the skin. Now, this is very important: *If you have tanned, olive, or black skin,* **run the other way.** IPL can cause discoloration that won't fade and will need to be treated for as long as six months. (Actually, fixing this problem is one of my specialties.)

— *What to expect:* Pigmented areas will get lighter with each treatment. How many you have will depend on your needs.

— *Know this:* Avoid sun exposure, tanning beds, and tanning products for four weeks before and after your treatment. The pulse will feel like the snap of a rubber band on the skin. The pigment in the treated area will typically get darker (like chocolate chips), become dry, and then flake off in four to seven days.

— *Estimated cost:* $250 to $400 per treatment.

TREATMENTS FOR PIGMENTATION

1. Cosmelan®

— *What it is:* Cosmelan is a depigmentation treatment program in the form of a mask that's applied at the clinic to the pigmented areas. The program works in tandem with an at-home cream used several times a day for a prescribed amount of time.

— *Who it's for:* It's great for people with melasma or "pregnancy masking" (excessive pigmentation caused by hormones). People with this condition cannot be treated with light-based treatments such as IPL because they exacerbate the problem. Cosmelan decreases dark patches by suppressing an enzyme in your skin that produces melanin. It also rejuvenates and smooths skin texture.

— *What to expect:* This is a long-term treatment that requires a home maintenance program. The cream is applied two or three times a day for the first two weeks, then once a day for up to six months. You will see some immediate improvement in pigmentation and improvement in texture in three to six weeks.

— *Know this:* You should not use products containing glycolic acid for a week before beginning treatment. You might get some reddening, slight itching, and flaking for a couple of days. If you don't protect yourself from the sun, discoloration can reappear.

— *Estimated cost:* $600 to $1,000, depending on the size of the area to be treated.

2. TCA Peel

— *What it is:* A trichloroacetic acid (TCA) peel is considered a medium-depth peel—it's more effective than a light peel and has less downtime than a deeper one. The chemical sloughs off the outer dead layer of skin. The TCA peel, which is safe for olive and light brown skins, is FDA approved.

— *Who it's for:* This is only for people with stubborn pigmentation problems such as melasma and severe sun damage. It's not as safe as lasers, which I prefer for minor sun damage and resurfacing.

— *What to expect:* After the peeling, your face will initially be red for up to two weeks; however, you'll then see an improvement in the color, freshness, and texture of your complexion. Results can last anywhere from six months to two years, and then you can have additional peels.

— *Know this:* Make sure to get your peel from a trained expert, because if done incorrectly, it can cause scarring. Whereas lasers are calibrated to operate at a certain skin depth, peels depend upon the skill of the technician performing them. And there are many factors that must be considered: The application of the acid can sting intensely for a few minutes. You will have approximately one week of downtime, where you most likely won't want to be in public. The outer layers of your skin will darken, crack, flake, and peel off (although this part is painless). You'll have to use ointment on your face during this time and avoid sun exposure. Never peel the skin off by force—allow it to flake off on its own.

— *Estimated cost:* $500 to $1,500, depending on the size of area to be treated.

HYFRECATOR (SKIN-GROWTH TREATMENT)

— *What it is:* A tiny probe using electrical currents at various settings. It's often used to shrink and seal blood vessels, although at my clinic, we prefer to use the less invasive laser for this issue. We do use this treatment on skin tags—those small, benign, flesh-colored growths that typically crop up in areas where clothing causes friction.

— *Who it's for:* Men who get skin tags in their neck area where their collar rubs, or women who get them where their bra hits.

— *What to expect:* The skin tags will disappear permanently, although if you're prone to this type of problem, you may get more of them.

— *Know this:* You should not take any blood thinners, aspirin, or drink alcohol for 72 hours before your treatment. This procedure can sting in sensitive areas, but you can have a topical painkiller. This is a quick procedure with no downtime.

— *Estimated cost:* $25 to $50 per spot.

VASCULAR THERAPY AND HAIR REMOVAL

I. CoolGlide Vascular Therapy

— *What it is:* This is a laser system that can be adjusted to target small areas. It cools the surface of the skin so as not to burn it. Then pulsed light energy causes blood to clot and destroys the small veins, which are then reabsorbed by your body.

— *Who it's for:* Anyone with small facial veins that have become more visible because the skin has gotten really thin and the veins have become more exposed. It's also great for cherry angiomas (small, benign, raised, and red skin tags) and rosacea.

— *What to expect:* On veins, it instantly works right before your eyes. It's amazing! You might need up to three treatments because veins can reroute themselves. Angiomas could scab and turn gray before fading away.

— *Know this:* You will feel a slight snap from the laser. In rare cases, there might be minor redness, swelling, or bruising. You should lay off vigorous exercise for 24 hours, and wear sun protection on treated areas.

— *Estimated cost:* Around $300 for every 15-minute treatment.

2. CoolGlide Laser Hair Removal

— *What it is:* A laser alternative to electrolysis or waxing, it can be used on all skin types and colors, including suntanned skin. It will not, however, work on gray or light blonde hair. By zapping hundreds of hair follicles at once, it's a much quicker option than electrolysis, which only targets one follicle at a time.

— *Who it's for:* This can be used on all skin types and is one of the only hair-removal systems that can be used on dark skin because it cools the skin's top layer.

— *What to expect:* It works on hair that is actively growing. Since hair is in different growth phases at any given time, you might need three to six treatments in one area to put all of the follicles out of action.

— *Know this:* You should not wax before the treatment because the laser is attracted to the hair follicle. However, you *should* shave so that the laser is not attracted to the dark pigment in the hair. You might feel a mild pinch from the laser. The treated area can be a bit red and swollen for a few hours.

— *Estimated cost:* $250 to $1,500, depending on the area.

3. Solera ProWave 770

— *What it is:* This is a flexible system that uses infrared light with three modes for working on various skin types and colors. However, it's not for patients with very dark skin. It, too, is a faster option than electrolysis.

— *Who it's for:* This is an IPL system, so it cannot be used on people with deep tans, chronic skin damage, or dark skin. On others, it permanently removes facial hair and is often used on larger areas such as the legs, back, and underarms.

— *What to expect:* For best results, you may need more than one treatment, and treatments are scheduled about six weeks apart.

— *Know this:* You cannot be treated if you've recently been in the sun. After treatment, you can be a little red and swollen for a while.

— *Estimated cost:* $150 to $1,500, depending on the area.

What Not to Do

There are so many excellent treatments on the market today. However, amid all of the excellent options out there, there are others that get a lot of hype, and I don't know why. There are a few well-known treatments that I generally don't like, don't believe in, and don't recommend. I've tried them—so have my clients—and I've had to correct the resulting damage or side effects. Of course, while my opinions are based on my professional experience, they are still my personal opinions.

Here are a few treatments (and prescriptions) I'd avoid:

— *Microdermabrasion.* This works by sanding your skin with aluminum-oxide crystals to "polish" it, and then suctioning the crystals up along with the abraded skin cells. The crystals inflict physical injury on your skin, which is just not made to take such a beating. The vacuuming can also break capillaries on the surface of the skin, creating redness or even pigmentation from the injury.

— *Radio frequency.* The idea behind this is to tighten collagen with heat, but when it first came out, it was going deeper than the collagen level and into the fat layer. It caused fat necrosis (basically melting), and the result was a waffling effect that looked a bit like cellulite on the face. The process has now been much improved, but I still think that there are better options available.

— *Oral antibiotics for acne.* Ingested antibiotics have systemic effects in that they can cause fungal or yeast infections and upset your digestive system. I always try to treat the inflammation and infection of acne with topicals and light treatments.

— *Accutane (isotretinoin).* I do everything in my power to keep my clients from going on Accutane. I know how painful acne can be, but this prescription drug can have serious side effects. Not only do you constantly have to get blood tests to make sure that your blood is healthy and your liver is safe while you're on it, but it may affect your mental health and who knows what else. There are too many options out there for acne today to choose something that may impact your overall health like this.

— *Cortisone shots for cystic acne.* I definitely don't recommend these, since they tend to degrade collagen and leave an indentation in the skin that's much worse than the blemish itself. The marks might not even appear until years later, once you've already done damage to your skin. Cortisone shots should only be used as a last resort.

— *Harsh acid peels.* These can be erratic in the way they penetrate the skin. In some spots they'll go down deep and in others they won't, so you get an uneven peel. Such peels can also be dangerous. I prefer the TCA peel.

— *Phenol peels.* Again, these are too harsh and too deep, and even one peel can be toxic to your liver.

— CO_2 *laser.* I don't recommend this because it's harsh and can leave your skin looking waxy and unnatural and cause a demarcation. Technology has changed, so you don't really need this treatment, although some skin-care practitioners still use it.

I know that these last several pages have given you a lot of information, but I've done my best to help edit the list and summarize what I think works best in each category. I hope that you'll use this chapter as a reference as you consider options for your particular skin type and goals.

Let's now break down two more important elements to skin health—products and ingredients.

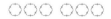

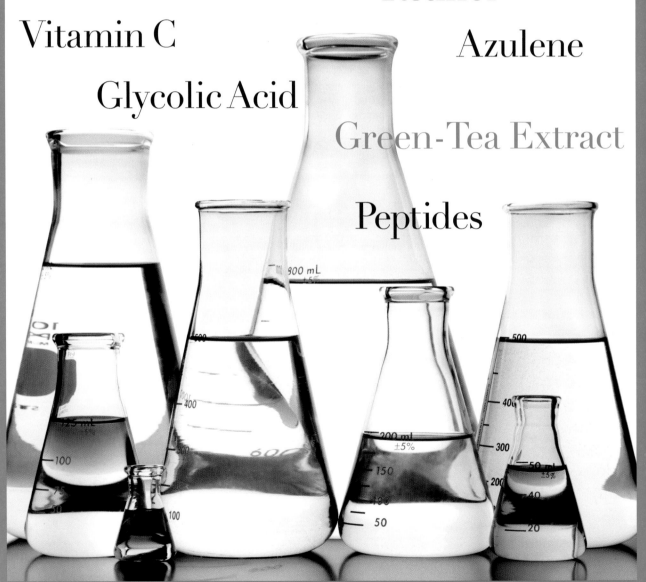

Matrixyl 3000

Alpha-Arbutin

Phytic Acid

Hyaluronic Acid

HSC Complex

Blue-Lotus Extract

Retinol

Vitamin C

Azulene

Glycolic Acid

Green-Tea Extract

Peptides

CHAPTER 7

Products and Ingredients That Deliver

We do a lot with treatments.
However, products are your personal tools—
your arsenal!—and are key to the improvement
and maintenance of your skin. And because of recent innovations
and discoveries, ingredients combined in thoughtful formulations
can dramatically change the health and state of your skin.

Products are the serums, lotions, creams, and medications you use topically. *Serums* are light, generally water based, and have delivery systems that take ingredients into the skin; your skin literally drinks them in. Because serums penetrate the layers of your skin so effectively, you often see results more rapidly and noticeably than with creams and lotions.

Moisturizing *creams* and *lotions* have waxes and oils in them that help them stay on top of your skin and seal it. But in recent years, the introduction of liposome technology has been a breakthrough in that it allows some creams to deliver certain ingredients farther down into the skin. Liposomes are something you may have read about; they're tiny "bubbles" that help a substance penetrate a cell. When they're used to encapsulate an ingredient in skin cream, for instance, they take that ingredient with them into the lower layers. There are a lot of exciting new possibilities for liposomes in the research stage. There may even come a time when we can target specific skin cells with treatments meant just for them.

The FDA will tell you that topical products only go so far. But try putting some peppermint oil on the bottoms of your feet—within minutes, you'll taste it in your mouth! So you do need to watch what you put on your skin. You really can transform your complexion through products when dealing with acne breakouts or certain textural concerns, such as dryness and pigmentation. For deeper issues, such as scarring and deep wrinkles, products are often combined with some of the treatments I mentioned in the last chapter for the best results.

What Are You Actually Putting on Your Face?

I have chemists coming to me every day with new ingredients, but I'm not going to use just anything on my clients or in my products. When something new comes out, know this: I read every study. I only use ingredients that have been thoroughly tested in a lab, and my team and I use them in the correct doses. And, most important, I learn how to put various components and ingredients together. After all, ingredients are only as good as the formulation.

You all know that there are so many ingredients on the market, and this book is not meant to be a cosmetic-chemistry dictionary. Instead, in this chapter I highlight those ingredients that stand out, perform, and are safe and effective when used correctly— and most of the ones I mention are those I use in my own products. I've listed what they are, what they do, how they work, and who they're for. Along with their common name,

I've also included the really long name chemists give them so that you'll know what to look for when you're shopping and reading labels.

I've categorized all of these topical ingredients into our Skin Health Pyramid levels: protect, hydrate, feed, stimulate, and detox. Some ingredients do double duty, and in those cases, I've put them into the category in which they primarily fit.

LEVEL 1: PROTECT

These are ingredients that protect your skin from UVA and UVB rays and other environmental damage; they help fight free radicals, too.

1. Physical Sun Barriers

— *What they are:* Physical sunscreens form a barrier on the skin's surface that deflects the damaging UV rays of the sun. They provide full-spectrum protection; in other words, they repel both UVA and UVB rays.

— *Who they're for:* Everyone.

— *What to expect:* Physical-barrier sunscreens are highly effective in protecting you from sun damage.

— *Know this:* You're probably familiar with the image of a beach lifeguard with a smear of white on his nose. That's zinc oxide, and that conspicuous color is the problem with barrier sunscreens. Manufacturers are now making much more refined products, but some brands with these properties still leave a slight whitish film on your face.

— *Look for:* Zinc, zinc oxide, Z-cote, titanium dioxide.

2. Chemical Sunscreens

— *What they are:* Chemical sunscreens absorb the UV rays before they reach your skin.

— *Who they're for:* Almost everyone, except for the supersensitive, who may react to the chemicals in them. People with oily skin will want to look for oil-free brands.

— *What to expect:* If used correctly, these type of sunscreens can protect you from the effects of the sun and aging. Look for full-spectrum brands that work against both UVA and UVB rays.

— *Know this:* Oil-based sunscreens can cause you to break out if you're prone to acne. These need to be applied 20 minutes before sun exposure. They should be applied last in your regimen and reapplied every three hours.

— *Look for:* Avobenzone, homosalate, octinoxate, octisalate, octocrylene, oxybenzone.

LEVEL 2: HYDRATE

These are the ingredients that provide a barrier to discourage evaporation from your skin, help pull moisture from the atmosphere into your cells, and seal in that moisture to keep you looking supple and youthful. This is the category where there really are a huge number of ingredients, and it can be particularly confusing. While it would be impossible to list every single one, those in this section will give you a good place to start.

1. Humectants

— *What they are:* Humectants are hydrators that attract moisture to your skin cells, and they increase the water content in the skin's top layers by drawing moisture from the surrounding air. They're derived from many sources, including desert plants and microorganisms.

— *Who they're for:* Everyone, since one of their jobs is to hydrate skin. It's that inability to hold water in our cells that causes many of the signs of aging, so we need humectant products to draw in moisture.

— *What to expect:* Hydrators plump up fine lines and wrinkles, giving your skin a smooth, youthful glow.

— *Know this:* You have to do your own research to find what hydrators work best for your skin type.

— *Look for:* Hyaluronic acid, sodium hyaluronate, glycerin, glycerides, propylene glycol, sorbitol, chondroitin sulphate, dermatan sulphate, urea, sesame-seed oil, pectins, colloidal oatmeal, honey, lecithin, polysaccharides.

2. Hyaluronic Acid

— *What it is:* You probably noticed this ingredient in the humectants section, but it's so important that I wanted to single it out and expand upon it. You see, hyaluronic acid is a substance found naturally in the human body that cushions and lubricates joints, eyes, and heart valves. Skin tissue has high concentrations of it, but it depletes as we age.

— *Who it's for:* Everyone. Since it's not oil based, it's good for people with acne or oily skin.

— *What it does:* It binds water, and one of its jobs is to hydrate collagen. Hyaluronic acid can hold a thousand times its weight in water in the cell, therefore delivering serious hydration!

— *What to expect:* Serums and creams with hyaluronic acid seal moisture on the skin and plump up fine lines and wrinkles, giving your skin a smooth, youthful glow.

— *Know this:* No side effects have been reported.

— *Look for:* Hyaluronic acid, sodium hyaluronate.

3. Occlusives

— *What they are:* Occlusives bind moisture to your skin and slow the loss of water by forming a barrier on the skin's surface. (Emollients, which are described next, can also act as occlusives.)

— *Who they're for:* Almost everyone, except for people with extremely oily skin. Those individuals with oily and/or acne-prone skin should avoid any substance that is pore clogging and comedogenic (that is, that promotes or aggravates acne).

— *What to expect:* Occlusives keep your skin feeling soft and smooth.

— *Know this:* There are no known side effects, but some people may be allergic to some ingredients.

— *Look for:* Beeswax, lecithin, dimethicone, ceramides, cetyl alcohol, grapeseed oil.

4. Emollients

— *What they are:* Emollients add lubrication to the surface of the skin. You may have heard the term *lipids.* Well, emollients are basically lipids—that is, fats and oils—that fill in the cracks between skin cells. If you think of your skin cells as bricks, lipids are fatty acids that form part of the mortar that holds them together.

— *Who they're for:* Just about everyone. Because they're fats, lipids prevent water from leaking through, so they have a moisturizing effect by binding water in your skin and preventing evaporation. They also improve the barrier function of the skin, rendering it less susceptible to bacteria, irritants, and the like.

— *What to expect:* Topically applied, emollients mimic the action of those naturally occurring in your skin. You should see smoother, plumper skin with regular use.

— *Know this:* There are no known side effects, but some people may be allergic to certain ingredients. You want to stick with those fats that are not hydrogenated and avoid trans fats (same as in your diet).

— *Look for:* Natural butters such as shea, avocado, açai, passion fruit, mango, coconut, and babassu; olive oil, rose-hip oil, evening-primrose oil, and the like; fatty acids such as omega-3 and omega-6; esters; ceramides; gamma-linolenic acid (GLA); squalane.

5. HSC Complex

— *What it is:* This is a complex that performs the functions of all of the aforementioned hydrating ingredients. However, it's also an advanced system that delivers and locks moisture in skin cells, restoring balance and replenishing skin lipids. I use this ingredient in three of my own products.

— *Who it's for:* Anyone who wants a dewy, glowing complexion, but especially those with very dry skin.

— *What to expect:* You'll see immediate results.

— *Know this:* There are no known side effects.

— *Look for:* HSC complex, glycosylceramides, sphingolipids, cyclomethicone, dimethiconol, octyl cocoate, phenyl trimethicone, ceramide 3, glycine soja (soyabean) sterol.

LEVEL 3: FEED

These are ingredients that feed the skin the nutrients you may not get from your food. You can apply them topically to fight free-radical damage and to calm, soothe, and heal skin.

1. Vitamin C

— *What it is:* This antioxidant is one of the most popular additives in cosmetic products, as well as one of the most researched.

— *Who it's for:* Those with pigmentation issues and anyone who wants healthier-looking skin (however, those with rosacea, active acne, and sensitive skin should avoid it). Vitamin C has been shown to protect skin from sun damage by reducing free radicals. Also, exposure to harmful UV rays decreases your skin's natural vitamin C levels, so topical vitamin C restores the protection you lose.

— *What to expect:* With consistent usage, you should see a reduction in fine lines and wrinkles and improved texture. Studies show that vitamin C may also boost collagen and brighten pigmentation over time.

— *Know this:* Vitamin C is really hard to stabilize and does not stay fresh for long. When any serum that contains vitamin C turns yellow, it's oxidized and should be thrown out. Not only is it no longer effective, but it can cause irritation and actually *increase* free radicals.

— *Look for:* Vitamin C, vitamin C complex, vitamin C ester, L-ascorbic acid, ascorbyl palmitate, sodium ascorbyl phosphate, retinyl ascorbate.

2. Vitamin E

— *What it is:* This is a plant-based, fat-soluble vitamin that is also a powerful antioxidant. It's a very common ingredient in skin-care products.

— *Who it's for:* Vitamin E is great for all skin types. It's important because it protects lipids from free-radical damage. When included in products, it's able to be absorbed by the skin and reach the living cells. It also protects against sun damage and even increases the effectiveness of sunscreens.

— *What to expect:* Because it's oil based, this vitamin really helps moisturize.

— *Know this:* It may clog pores, so you might want to avoid this ingredient if you're prone to breakouts.

— *Look for:* Alpha-tocopheryl acetate, tocopheryl linoleate, tocotrienols, and/or tocopheryl succinate.

3. Alpha-Lipoic Acid

— *What it is:* This versatile antioxidant that your body makes naturally is exceptional because it fights a wide range of free radicals. It also works in conjunction with vitamins C and E, making them more effective. Also, it can reach both water- and oil-based areas of the skin.

— *Who it's for:* Everyone, especially those who are aging. One of its important jobs is to protect the components of DNA that degrade as we age.

— *What to expect:* Since it promotes energy in living cells and helps with the exfoliation of dead cells, alpha-lipoic acid promotes a healthy glow.

— *Know this:* It appears to be safe for almost everyone.

— *Look for:* Alpha-lipoic acid or thioctic acid.

4. Green-Tea Extract

— *What it is:* Green tea may be nature's most potent antioxidant. It contains a phytonutrient called EGCG that has been quite widely studied and shown to eradicate free radicals. I use it throughout my product line.

— *Who it's for:* Everyone. Green tea helps promote elasticity and may enhance sun protection (when used along with sunscreen). It can also aid in the reduction of rosacea and inflammation. In addition, one study showed that it can help with mild acne.

— *What to expect:* You likely will see an even skin tone, soothed irritation, and reduction in redness.

— *Know this:* It's uncommon, but some people are allergic to tea.

— *Look for:* Green-tea extract, camellia sinensis.

5. Botanical Extracts

— *What they are:* Increasingly, chemists are tapping into the world of plants to find ingredients to feed your face. There is a wealth of botanicals from all over the globe being incorporated into products these days.

— *Who they're for:* More and more people don't want to use products derived from animal sources or that are chemically manufactured. These ingredients offer an effective alternative for them . . . and the rest of us.

— *What to expect:* Ingredients that can play a variety of roles in boosting the efficacy of products.

— *Know this:* Most botanicals have a long history of safe usage in folk medicine. However, some people might have allergies to certain plants.

— *Look for:* Camellia sinensis (tea) extract, rosmarinus officinalis (rosemary) extract, nymphaea coerulea (blue lotus) extract, boerhavia diffusa (red spiderling) extract, epilobium angustifolium (fireweed or Canadian willowherb) extract, lavender extract, cucumis sativus (cucumber) extract.

6. Aloe Vera

— *What it is:* It's an African succulent plant.

— *Who it's for:* Everyone, unless you have a known allergy. Aloe-vera gel has powerful soothing properties, and it's great for both individuals with oily skin and those with eczema and rosacea. People also use it for treating sunburns, as it appears to speed healing.

— *What to expect:* Soothing, moisturizing, and healing effects.

— *Know this:* It has a centuries-long history of safe usage as a natural remedy for minor burns and wounds.

— *Look for:* Aloe vera, aloe barbadensis extract.

When it comes to ingredients, stimulants are those that provoke the skin to perform a different function: for example, peptides ask it to produce more collagen and elastin, while brighteners ask it to reduce melanin production. These are the products that induce your skin to turn back the clock so that you don't have lines and wrinkles or discoloration.

I. Vitamin A

— *What it is:* The type of vitamin A used topically is known as retinol and is found in many cosmetic brands. Retin-A is a stronger, prescription version of retinol, and it's amazing—it can transform your skin.

— *Who it's for:* For people who are aging, retinol has the ability to penetrate skin to speed up cell turnover and stimulate collagen. Studies have shown that it helps resurface and rejuvenate the skin by reducing fine lines and wrinkles, rough patches, and hyperpigmentation. It's also effective for acne, scarring, enlarged pores, and textural issues.

— *What to expect:* Retin-A works very quickly on signs of aging. However, when you first start using it, you'll go through what I call the skin-cleansing phase, where cells turn over a lot, and you're going to be red and flaky. (You can dissolve that top layer away with a gentle exfoliant.) As you continue using the product, your skin gets used to it, so you won't continue to have the surface dryness and peeling. In addition, you can use it all the way up to your eye area and down your neck and chest.

I've had many clients in their 50s who started using Retin-A when they were in their 30s, and I have to say that their skin looks healthier and younger than those who didn't use it, or those who didn't start until much later.

— *Know this:* Vitamin A products can be irritating, leaving your skin red and peeling. You may notice sensitivity around the mucous membranes near the nose and mouth, so avoid those areas. Introduce these products into your regimen gradually instead of blasting your skin with them every day, otherwise you'll just end up with a peeling, red mess. If you are acne prone, select a gel-based form.

At our clinic, we tell clients who are really sensitive to mix a pea-sized amount of vitamin A products in with their moisturizer three times a week. I also tell people not to use them before a big event. (If you're pregnant or breast-feeding, you shouldn't use them at all.) And do be sure to apply sun protection when using them.

— *Look for:* Vitamin A, retinol, retinoic acid, tretinoin, retinyl palmitate, retinyl actate. Prescription brands include: Retin-A, Atralin, Renova, Avita, Altinac.

2. Peptides

— *What they are:* Peptides are chains of amino acids that are the building blocks of collagen. There are a number of peptide additives in cosmetics. One of the most effective compounds is Matrixyl 3000 (palmitoyl-tripeptide and palmitoyl-oligopeptide), which has been shown in studies to boost collagen *and* hyaluronic acid.

— *Who they're for:* Peptides are messengers that communicate between our epidermis and dermis. As we get older, this exchange becomes less efficient, and collagen production declines as a result. Topically applied peptides boost collagen production by leading the dermis into thinking that it's sent a lot of collagen to the surface and should make more.

— *What to expect:* With consistent use, a reduction in fine lines and wrinkles and younger-looking skin. There has been a clinical study that showed that using Matrixyl 3000 reduced deep wrinkles by 45 percent after two months.

— *Know this:* You must get the maximum dosage of peptides in order for them to work. They are very expensive, and any product that claims to have peptides but is bargain priced probably doesn't have enough to be effective. Plus, peptides need a good "delivery" system such as liposomes to take them down into the skin.

— *Look for:* Brand names Matrixyl and Dermaxyl; terms such as acetyl hexapeptide-3, palmitoyl-oligopeptide, palmitoyl tetrapeptide-7.

3. Neuropeptides

— *What they are:* Types of peptides that are released by the brain and found naturally in your body. In cosmetics, certain neuropeptides act a little bit like topical Botox: they relax facial muscle contractions that cause lines and furrows, especially on your forehead, around your eyes, and above your lips.

— *Who they're for:* People with expression lines and wrinkling.

— *What to expect:* You'll start to see results in wrinkle reduction after 15 days, and even more by day 30.

— *Know this:* There are no known side effects. However, for a neuropeptide to work, you need to get products that have at least a 5 percent solution of the ingredient.

— *Look for:* Argireline, acetyl hexapeptide-3.

4. Kojic Acid

— *What it is:* Kojic acid is a natural substance that's made from fungi. It's a by-product of making sake in Japan.

— *Who it's for:* People with hyperpigmentation from sun damage, melasma or the so-called pregnancy mask, and freckles.

— *What to expect:* Kojic acid can produce good results in evening out skin tone.

— *Know this:* When exposed to light and air, it can degrade and become less effective. For that reason, some cosmetic companies use the more stable kojic dipalmitate instead, although it's less potent.

— *Look for:* Kojic acid, kojic dipalmitate.

5. Licorice Extract

— *What it is:* Recently, scientists discovered that glabridin, an extract from the licorice plant, is a powerful skin brightener. It works by suppressing the formation of melanin.

— *Who it's for:* People with hyperpigmentation and melasma. It also has anti-inflammatory properties, so it's a good choice for sensitive or acne-prone skin.

— *What to expect:* Studies have shown that some people start to see effects within a week, but you won't note the full results until the top layer of skin cells has been replaced.

— *Know this:* Licorice has been used medicinally in Europe for centuries.

— *Look for:* Licorice extract, glabridin.

6. Hydroquinone

— *What it is:* Hydroquinone has been the most commonly used skin lightener for some time. That's because it doesn't bleach skin but disrupts the production of melanin that causes hyperpigmentation.

— *Who it's for:* It is extremely effective in lightening areas of pigmented or darkened skin such as freckles, age spots, and melasma.

— *What to expect:* You'll see pigment lightening very quickly. Even so, it's more effective if it's massaged into the skin, to help the product penetrate.

— *Know this:* Hydroquinone can cause drying, burning, irritation, redness, and peeling. You need to stay out of the sun when using it, and may notice increased sensitivity to other topical products. Avoid it if you're pregnant. This should be used as a spot treatment only and for short-term use. It comes in different concentrations: 0.5 percent to 2 percent is sold over the counter; 4 percent and above is by pre-scription only.

Please note that hydroquinone has been banned in some European countries because of a cancer risk and is under review by the FDA, which is considering banning it in the U.S. as well.

— *Look for:* Hydroquinone.

LEVEL 5: DETOX

Everything in this section helps detoxify by cleansing, exfoliating, and ridding the skin of the top, dead layers of cells and increasing cell turnover; this then allows the other ingredients listed in this chapter to penetrate better and work more effectively. Some of these products are also very effective in ridding the skin of acne-causing agents, a crucial component to fighting breakouts.

I. Foaming Cleansers

— *What they are:* "Soapy" cleansers with ingredients that make them foam up. The most common ones contain sodium lauryl sulfate and sodium laureth sulfate and are basically detergents.

— *Who they're for:* Those prone to oiliness. They are also useful when you need to remove oil-based makeup.

— *What to expect:* Foaming cleansers are excellent for getting rid of surface dirt and oil.

— *Know this:* They can be too harsh for people with mature, dry, or sensitive skin; or for individuals with conditions such as rosacea and eczema.

— *Look for:* Sodium lauryl sulfate (or SLS), sodium laureth sulfate (or SLES).

2. Gel/Cream Cleansers

— *What they are:* These are sulfate-free cleansers that use other types of milder, less-drying, "sudsing" ingredients. They don't strip the skin as much, so the barrier function is not as compromised.

— *Who they're for:* Those with dry, mature, or sensitive skin; or those with eczema or rosacea.

— *What to expect:* They are equally effective for cleaning your skin but don't remove oil as well as foaming cleansers do.

— *Know this:* Because gel and cream cleansers are less aggressive, you may need to wash twice to get all of the makeup and debris off of the skin.

— *Look for:* Sodium C14-16 olefin sulfonate, disodium oleamido mea sulfosuccinate, oleyl betaine.

3. Glycolic Acid

— *What it is:* A strong AHA (alpha hydroxy acid) derived from sugar cane, although it can also be made synthetically. Glycolic acid works very fast to turn over skin cells by weakening the lipids that glue dead skin cells together, which allows those cells to slough off. It also draws moisture to the skin.

— *Who it's for:* Anyone who can take a fairly strong, superficial peel. It's not re-commended for those with very thin skin.

— *What to expect:* This ingredient has changed skin care because it really works. It's also a great multitasker that improves a lot of skin issues, including fine lines, dullness, pigmentation, and enlarged pores.

— *Know this:* Glycolic acid was a major breakthrough in the skin-care industry, but I think it's overused. I feel that too much glycolic actually breaks down collagen, so I recommend using small doses once or twice a week—do not use it as a daily moisturizer!

When buying glycolic products, you have to consider the strength *and* the pH level. Strengths in over-the-counter products vary all the way from 3 to 40 percent, and because studies have shown that increasing the pH also makes glycolic more effective, you shouldn't buy anything with a pH level lower than 3.5. Do be sure to use a sunblock, since you can become more sensitive to ultraviolet rays.

— *Look for:* Glycolic acid.

4. Lactic Acid

— *What it is:* A natural AHA made mostly from milk—but can also be made from cornstarch, potatoes, or molasses—lactic acid is gentler than glycolic acid and doesn't penetrate as deeply. It accelerates cell turnover and helps with the moisturization of upper cell layers by increasing product penetration.

— *Who it's for:* This ingredient is great for people who are really sensitive, or even those who are prone to allergies. It's one of my personal favorites because I'm very sensitive.

— *What to expect:* Lactic acid is effective for acne; you'll also see improvement in a number of other skin problems, including wrinkles, discoloration, and psoriasis. Because it's gentle, you'll get the best results after about three months. The key to it is a special trick I learned: You should soak a pad and then gently buff the skin with it, back and forth in tiny motions. You can get rid of that top layer of skin this way.

— *Know this:* Even though lactic acid is not as strong as glycolic acid, the same caveats about pH levels and using protection from the sun still apply.

— *Look for:* Lactic acid.

5. Phytic Acid

— *What it is:* A less commonly used acid made from nuts, seeds, cereal grains, and legumes. It's a newer ingredient in the skin-care world, but I happen to love it and its antioxidant properties.

— *Who it's for:* Phytic acid is great for people with acne—it acts as an exfoliator but is much gentler than glycolic acid. It's also an effective lightening agent and acts as a melanin blocker. As a matter of fact, it's a key ingredient in my anti-acne line.

— *What to expect:* After about three months, a reduction in acne scars and a more even skin tone.

— *Know this:* As with all AHAs, you should use sunblock.

— *Look for:* Phytic acid.

6. Salicylic Acid

— *What it is:* The most common BHA (beta hydroxy acid) used in skin care today. Where AHAs are only water soluble, BHAs are also oil soluble.
Salicylic acid is derived from plants and related to aspirin. And like aspirin, it has anti-inflammatory properties. It also softens keratin, a protein that forms part of the skin structure—this helps loosen dry and scaly skin, making it easier to remove. Along with being an effective exfoliant, this acid also strips away oil and cleanses pores.

— *Who it's for:* It a good option for people with acne or for oily skin types.

— *What to expect:* Salicylic acid shows great results for acne and oily skin.

— *Know this:* It can be really drying. You also have to be careful if you're allergic to aspirin, since you may be allergic to this acid as well. It can also increase sun sensitivity, so do wear sunblock.

— *Look for:* Salicylic acid, SA125P, 2-hydroxy benzoic acid.

7. Fruit Enzymes

— *What they are:* These are natural "chemicals" from fruit, primarily pineapple, papaya, and pumpkin. They're all protein-digesting enzymes, which means that when applied topically, they "eat" dead skin cells. I love to combine fruit enzymes with fine grains because then you get physical exfoliation combined with chemical exfoliation.

— *Who they're for:* Anyone who wants a gentle exfoliator. In medicine, pineapple has been employed to help heal burns and papaya has been used for wound healing.

— *What to expect:* Immediate results that leave your skin smooth and fresh. Long term, you may see an improvement in brown spots and fine lines.

— *Know this:* A small number of people are allergic to these substances, so stop using them if you get rashes or irritation.

— *Look for:* Bromelain (pineapple), papain (papaya), cucurbito pepo fruit ferment extract (pumpkin).

8. Topical Antibiotics

— *What they are:* These are prescription topical medications that usually come in a solution, gel, lotion, or ointment. They kill acne-causing bacteria and reduce infections in the pores.

— *Who they're for:* Those with moderate to severe acne in the form of cysts, whiteheads, or clogged pores. They're also sometimes prescribed for acne rosacea.

— *What to expect:* You should notice a decrease in breakouts.

— *Know this:* Topical antibiotics can be very irritating and drying. I generally don't like using them to treat acne because there are too many other safe and effective options. In rare cases, however, I recommend using them to jump-start the healing process and kill infection (usually for those with severe acne). Just understand that if used for prolonged periods, they may stop working. They also leave skin very photosensitive, so always wear sunscreen when using them.

— *Look for:* Clindamycin, erythromycin, metronidazole (for acne rosacea).

9. Topical Steroids

— *What they are:* These are usually prescription topical medications (also known as corticosteroids) that come in many forms, including sprays, gels, lotions, or ointments. They are chemical compounds that reduce inflammation.

— *Who they're for:* Those who have extreme rashes or dryness, or individuals with severe cases of eczema or psoriasis.

— *What to expect:* These topicals will reduce inflammation and redness in addition to calming rashes and suppressing eczema or psoriasis outbreaks.

— *Know this:* I only advocate the use of steroids in extreme cases and in limited doses. Steroids can thin the skin and compromise its immune function. Prolonged use can cause other health issues, including the suppression of the body's natural steroid production. In emergencies, I recommend steroids for severe rashes or stubborn outbreaks of eczema. The recommended use is three times a day for no more than five days. Be aware that there are seven classes (strengths) of steroids—class one is the highest, and class seven is the lowest—and different parts of the skin require different strengths.

— Look for: Hydrocortisone, clobetasone butyrate, clobetasol propionate, triamcinolone acetonide.

10. Benzoyl Peroxide

— What it is: It's a strong chemical that has been used for treating acne since the 1920s (albeit in a diluted form). In the form of gels, creams, cleansers, ointments, or pads, it's still the basic ingredient of many acne products on the market. I strongly recommend that you try to find a timed-release version because it won't give you a blast of irritation.

— Who it's for: Benzoyl peroxide is an antibacterial that kills germs by oxygenating the skin, so it's very effective for acne. It also helps soften and shed dead cells.

— What to expect: It has good results on mild to moderate acne, but it can be drying and irritating. The mildest solution of 2.5 percent is as effective as stronger solutions, but it's less drying.

— Know this: Even mild solutions of this chemical can cause extreme flaking and irritation. You should protect yourself from sunlight while using it.

— Look for: Benzoyl peroxide.

11. Sulfur

— What it is: Sulfur is a naturally occurring element that's been used for centuries to treat skin conditions.

— Who it's for: Anyone with serious congestion and breakouts. Sulfur helps shed dead skin cells and reduce clogged pores. It also has antimicrobial properties, so it inhibits the growth of bacteria.

— What to expect: Sulfur is great when used in the form of a mask or spot treatment and is very effective in drying up blemishes.

— *Know this:* Generally drying, it will cause skin to lightly flake. Use the product at night, and no more than a few days in a row to avoid irritation. Some people may experience a mild allergy, but most just don't like the smell!

— *Look for:* Sulfur, sulphur.

12. Tea-Tree Oil

— *What it is:* Distilled from the leaves of the melaleuca plant, this is one of the few essential oils that can be applied directly to the skin.

— *Who it's for:* People with mild acne. But tea-tree oil is very effective for many other conditions and works to fight bacterial and fungal infections, including toenail fungi. It also helps minimize oil production and kill acne-causing bacteria in the skin and is even good for healing cold sores and burns.

— *What to expect:* It has a fresh scent and can be applied directly to the blemish or oily region. It will help balance the skin and will eventually dry up a pimple, generally without causing irritation.

— *Know this:* Tea-tree oil is safe for most people. In fact, it has been used for years by the indigenous people of Australia.

— *Look for:* Tea-tree oil, melaleuca alternifolia.

13. Witch Hazel

— *What it is:* A mild, natural toner and antioxidant that's been around for centuries, witch hazel is also used as a versatile treatment for skin conditions such as bruises and hives. It comes from a small bush that's native to North America.

— *Who it's for:* Since it's gentle, witch hazel can be used on acne sufferers with sensitive skin.

— *What to expect:* Dabbed on a couple of times a day, it can reduce inflammation and soothe irritation.

— *Know this:* Although witch-hazel tea is a traditional Native American remedy, commercial extracts of witch hazel are not recommended for internal use.

— *Look for:* Witch hazel, hamamelis virginiana.

14. Mineral/Clay Masks

— *What they are:* Masks of natural materials. Mineral masks are formed by the weathering of certain minerals and tend to be both absorbent and toning. Clays are derived from various earths.

— *Who they're for:* People with oily and/or acne-prone skin, or those with sensitive skin. Minerals can be good for all skin types, including dry skin, but clay masks will be too drying for them.

— *What to expect:* Mineral masks are effective in the removal of excess sebum and dirt, while at the same time assisting in balancing oil production and calming the complexion. Clay masks will pull impurities and excess oil out of the pores.

— *Know this:* They are a gentle option for sensitive, oily skin and can help heal blemishes.

— *Look for:* Kaolin, aluminum silicate, silt, bentonite clay.

◇◇◇

Please know that most of the ingredients in this chapter really only work when they contain an effective dosage, which is the amount that was tested in trials. It's exactly the same as medication: if the doctor prescribes you 500 mg of some antibiotic but you only take 50 mg, it's not going to kill the infection. So before you spend a lot of money on a product, try to ascertain from the company's labeling or Website just how much of the desired ingredient is contained.

What to Avoid

As is the case with certain treatments, there are also ingredients that you should use with caution or avoid altogether. The following is a short list of the ones to watch out for:

— *Synthetic fragrances:* Many synthetic fragrances contain phthalates, which have been found to disrupt hormones. While they're especially high in products such as nail polish, they're also found in skin care. Whenever possible, my company tries to use essential oils for fragrance in our products.

— *Petrochemicals:* There is quite a long list of these, the most common being petrolatum, mineral oil, and paraffin. Most of them don't allow the skin to breathe— they clog pores and are therefore highly comedogenic.

— *Animal testing:* My company doesn't test products on animals, and I think it's important to avoid businesses and products that do. There are so many other, kinder ways to prove that products are safe and effective without resorting to these means.

— *Nanoparticles:* The jury is still out on these guys. Nanoparticles are tiny molecules that are able to deliver ingredients below the skin's surface, but they've also been found to penetrate even deeper tissue. Until more research is done, it's best to avoid them until their long-term effects are better understood.

◇◇◇

Now that you know what to look for when it comes to products and ingredients, let's talk a little about what else is out there. In addition to using products with great ingredients, there's a wealth of things you can do for your skin in the comfort of your very own home.

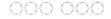

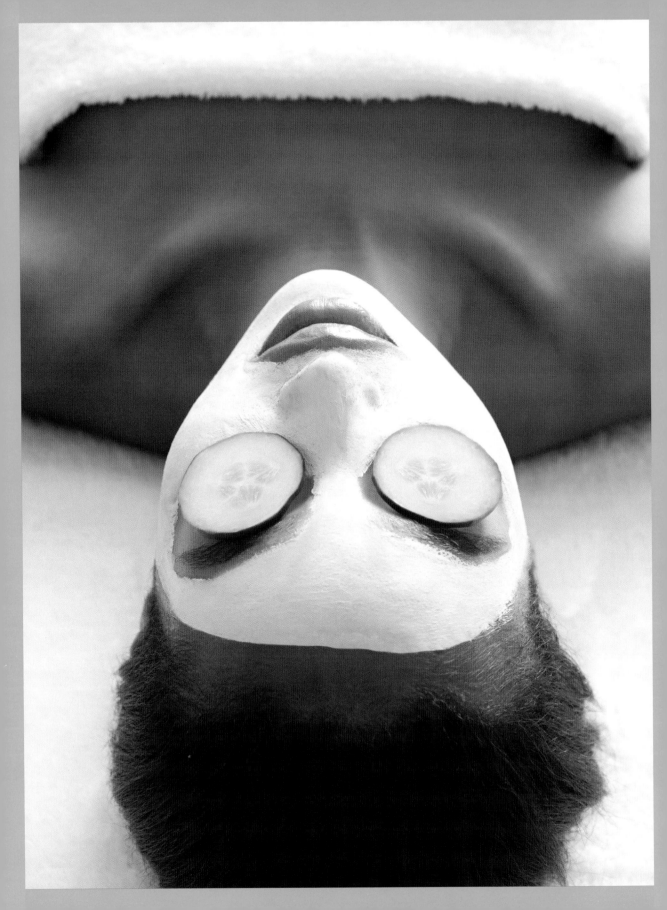

CHAPTER 8

At-Home Regimens That Work

When I first started in skin care, you couldn't get me out of my kitchen. I was constantly in there, concocting the latest remedies and testing them out on myself and my friends. To this day, I still love doing this. I'll apply an egg mask before a photo shoot, using the whites to tighten and firm my complexion. Sometimes I'll add goat's milk to the bath when my skin is irritated or when my eczema flares up.

Bringing It Home

Journalists are always asking me for tips and tricks and any special things that can be done with what's inside the fridge, cupboard, or medicine cabinet. I understand that treatments and products can get expensive, and they're not within everyone's budget. So while you may not get the exact same results you would from more costly in-office technologies, you'll still witness visible results with these affordable solutions. And the truth is, this is fun! It can be done during a relaxing night at home or in preparation for a night out.

In this chapter, I'm going to share some of my favorite fixes you can mix up at home. I'm also going to let you know what you should be doing daily for your skin. I'll detail an at-home regimen and even give you a step-by-step guide to give yourself a Kate Somerville facial, in the comfort of your home. I'll even give you tips on how to customize it, like we do in the clinic, for your particular skin type.

This chapter is pretty simple and straightforward, but I firmly believe that sticking to a daily routine will result in better skin now and as you age. I promise.

Morning Routine

STEP I: CLEANSE

Cleansing is key for healthy skin and is a crucial step. However, cleansing should be customized to your skin type, and you should select your cleanser with care:

- If you have dry or sensitive skin, just splash warm water on your face or use a gentle gel cleanser that does not contain sulfates.

- If you're oily or acne prone, cleansing with a salicylic-acid-based cleanser is a good option.

- For those of you who wear a lot of makeup, you may want to use a cleansing brush, or wash your skin twice.

STEP 2: EXFOLIATE

Do this one to three times a week, depending on skin type; if you get very red, try it at night:

- For delicate skin types and those with active acne, I recommend exfoliating once a week.

- For oily or combination skin, or if you have any discoloration, you may exfoliate up to three times a week.

Skin Care Brush, which we use in our clinic. It's a cleansing and exfoliation system that gently removes makeup and bacteria, and leaves skin incredibly smooth.

I find this to be a very exciting time—in the next few years, you'll definitely see more and more sophisticated technology that will turn your bathroom into your personal skin-care clinic. And just know that I am working very hard to bring our products and services home to you!

STEP 3: TREAT

Depending on your skin type, you'll want to feed it based on its particular needs:

- If you have sun damage and hyperpigmentation, you'll want to apply an antioxidant serum that will lighten spots and fight free radicals.

- If you have oily skin, you may want to apply a toner to reduce sebum production, or try a bacteria-busting treatment serum.

STEP 4: HYDRATE/MOISTURIZE

Regardless of skin type, it's key to deliver water to the cells and then seal it in, so skin absolutely glows with health:

- If you're oily or acne prone, make sure that the serums you use to deliver ingredients to your skin cells are in a water base.

- Remember that your lips are important, too. Use a lip balm that doesn't contain peppermint essential oils or petroleum, as both can actually dry out lips.

- Don't forget your neck and chest!

STEP 5: PROTECT

Apply an ample amount of sunscreen over your moisturizer.

Afternoon Routine

— Freshen up your look midday by spritzing a little water on your skin.

— If you're really oily, add a drop of tea-tree oil to the water. This should help control excess oil without your needing to reapply makeup.

— If you're in and out all day, you should reapply your sunscreen every couple of hours, or lightly dust on another layer of mineral makeup.

Skin-telligence:

PEACH-FUZZ FACE. There's no pretty way to say this: if you have a face full of fuzz and you aren't a piece of fruit, go ahead and shave. Generally, laser hair removal can't treat this fine and furry light-colored hair. Shaving will not only get rid of it efficiently, but you'll also get the added benefit of healthy exfoliation. And no, it won't grow back thicker or darker— this is an old wives' tale. Hair growth only changes because of hormonal fluctuations, usually an increase in testosterone.

Evening Routine

STEP 1: CLEANSE

Don't just use water in the evenings. Instead, go with a cleanser that's appropriate for your skin type:

- If you have oily or acne-prone skin and wear makeup, use a foaming cleanser to rid skin of debris.

- If you're dry, stick with a gentle gel cleanser.

STEP 2: EXFOLIATE

If you tend to have blemished, sensitive, or thin skin, I recommend exfoliating at night rather than during the day. Most forms of exfoliation can leave skin a little red, as they are stimulating.

STEP 3: TREAT

You'll want to treat the skin with repairing serums at night. Because our bodies are at rest, they tend to have more energy to heal and repair during this downtime:

- If you're acne prone, it's important to treat your skin with bacteria-fighting agents at night so that you'll wake up with clearer skin.

STEP 4: HYDRATE/MOISTURIZE

This step is very important in the evening, in order to replenish hydration lost during the day and during the cleansing process:

- Seal the serums and nutrients into your skin cells with a moisturizer. If you're especially dry, you can add a few drops of olive or rose-hip oil to your moisturizer.

- Pat on an eye cream to deliver important nutrition and age-defying ingredients and brighteners while your eyes are at rest.

- Moisturize your lips as well—you'll wake up in the morning with a smoother, plumper pout.

I've Got the Remedy—and So Do You

Homemade treatments can be very effective. Just remember: whenever you use natural ingredients or ingredients from your fridge, you should always do a little patch test on your skin first. This way, you'll make sure that you aren't too sensitive and won't react with an allergy or irritation.

Here are a few home remedies to treat some common concerns:

LIGHTENERS AND BRIGHTENERS

— *Aspirin treatment:* Aspirin contains acetylsalicylic acid, a salicylic-acid derivative. As we've already learned, salicylic acid is a very useful ingredient in combating acne, and it can also lighten pigmentation over time. If you have those issues, why not try this treatment once a week?

Heat up a few teaspoons of water. Add two whole aspirin tablets to the water, mash with a spoon, and mix thoroughly. Massage the mixture onto the skin and leave on for about five minutes. Repeated use of this treatment will lighten and brighten the skin over time.

— *Strawberry swipe:* Cut a large strawberry in half lengthwise. Take a fork and poke at the flesh a little to awaken and release the juices. Swipe the strawberry across your face, and massage the juice in a bit, using small circles. Leave it on for about two minutes and then rinse off with water. Strawberry juice contains natural skin lighteners that brighten spots over time.

You can also do the "strawberry swipe" a few times a week on your teeth for a gentle and safe teeth whitener!

— *Cucumber cooler:* Grab a cucumber from the fridge and slice it into thin slices. Lie down and carefully place them on your face. The cucumber will reduce redness and swelling and calm any sensitivities.

— *Ice device:* If you ever get out of the shower and are pretty red or notice that your pores appear large, try this: Soak a washcloth in an ice bath for a few minutes. Take the washcloth out, wring out the excess water, and lay the cloth across your face for about five minutes. You'll notice that your skin instantly looks much healthier and more refreshed. The cool temperature will also help close down pores and tighten the capillaries that cause redness.

The At-Home Facial

I believe in the power of an at-home facial, when done properly, for all skin types. It can leave your skin looking clear, healthy, and radiant; and your spirit renewed. And if you don't have the time or the cash to go to a salon or clinic, this is a great alternative.

The home facial is a staple of my personal regimen, and I do one every Sunday night. I get all of my tools ready, sit at my bathroom sink, and relax. It's "me" time!

Skin-telligence:

KITCHEN CHEMIST. If you run out of eye-makeup remover, look to your kitchen for the solution. Olive or grapeseed oil can be very effective for this purpose. These gentle oils break down the solids in mascara and nourish the delicate eye area at the same time. I also believe the oil helps condition the lashes and makes them grow longer and stronger, adding a little love to your lid!

I encourage you to enjoy this wonderful weekly ritual as well. First, gather some tools:

- A bottle of distilled or spring water
- A large bowl (it can be a family-sized salad bowl)
- Essential oils, depending on your skin type (see pages 137 and 138)
- A washcloth and hand towel
- A box of tissues
- A mild toner like witch hazel
- An antibiotic cream like Neosporin
- A few cotton balls
- A facial brush or fan brush (you can pick one up at an art-supply store)
- A standing mirror

Now get your products together:

- Cleanser
- Exfoliant
- Mask
- Treatment serum
- Moisturizer
- Eye cream

Next, I suggest that you read through all seven steps of the at-home facial to see what you're going to be doing. Once you feel comfortable with them, let's get started!

STEP 1: CLEANSE

Get rid of all of the makeup, dirt, debris, and other junk that's gathered on your skin. Use your favorite cleanser or try these:

— *Milk or heavy-cream wash:* Dip a cotton ball in heavy cream or milk and use it to cleanse your face. The lactose enzymes dissolve the dirt and debris, and the milk proteins nourish the skin.

— *Grape wash:* Muddle a few grapes and massage the flesh in circles across your face. This is a really simple and quick way to cleanse the skin.

STEP 2: STEAM

At my clinic, my staff and I always use steam at the beginning of our facial treatments, and I absolutely love doing it at home. Steam opens pores and releases impurities, and it also softens the skin and helps detach dead cells.

Fill the big bowl you gathered with the spring or distilled water, ensuring that it's hot enough to be steaming. Place two drops of essential oil in the water—this will not only provide extra skin benefits, but it will offer aromatherapy benefits as well.

Depending on your skin type, choose from these options:

- **Normal:** Lavender, which is generally pleasing to most individuals and relaxing to the mind.

- **Dry:** Chamomile is soothing and calms the nerves. Sandalwood is highly effective in balancing dehydration.

- **Sensitive/Rosacea/Eczema:** Chamomile is soothing and helps regenerate tissue. Cedarwood is known for its sedating qualities and ability to relieve itching.

- **Oily:** Ylang-ylang helps control oil production. Bergamot has antiseptic properties and can also reduce oiliness.

- **Combination:** Geranium is highly effective in both balancing the skin and the mind.

- **Acne:** Tea tree stimulates the immune system and is antibacterial and antifungal.

- **Scarring/Hyperpigmented:** Neroli, which has an incredible smell and re-generative properties for the skin, can help prevent and improve scarring.

- **Mature:** Sandalwood helps soften skin and improve the dehydration associated with aging.

- **Mature and Acne:** Chamomile reduces inflammation associated with acne and aging. Neroli promotes smoother skin and regeneration.

Place your face above the bowl of hot water for two to three minutes. The steam will help open your pores, releasing impurities and dead skin cells from the surface of your skin. You can also place a washcloth in the warm water, wring it out, and then lay it over your face for two to three minutes.

STEP 3: EXFOLIATE

Please don't select scrubs with ground-up nutshells—when crushed, these nuts are pretty jagged and can actually cause tiny tears on the surface of your skin. Those tears will then appear as sensitivity or irritation, and may also serve as little reservoirs for bacteria to attach and thrive. Ideally, you should be looking for scrubs with enzymes, acids, or round beads that *gently* roll across the surface and lift away dead skin cells.

If you have rosacea or eczema or your skin is broken out, please take extra caution when exfoliating. Choose a mild product that does not ablate the skin, and do the most delicate form of exfoliation so that you don't inflame your condition. Fruit enzymes are usually fine, but you can also try the following, which is gentle enough for most skin types:

— *Yogurt mask:* Apply about a teaspoon of plain, organic yogurt to your face and leave on for about five minutes. The lactose in the yogurt will gently dissolve the dead skin cells and leave your skin looking polished and feeling smooth.

STEP 4: EXTRACTIONS

Snap, crackle, *pop!* Believe it or not, it's okay to "pop a zit" (gasp!) *if you do it right.* I know that many people will disagree with me . . . but since you're probably doing it on your own anyway, you might as well do it correctly. After all, we facialists do this every day.

There's an art to extracting blackheads and whiteheads. While whiteheads eventually go away, blackheads are stubborn and will stay lodged in pores until they're physically cleansed. So it's important to know how to set your pores free.

The incorrect way to do extractions is to use your dirty fingernails and just squeeze away. When you try to pop a pimple without giving it a "canal," you're actually breaking the skin and creating an injury, which can leave a scar. The blemish can also erupt under the skin, which can lead to an infection. This is why it's important to use lancets. These short, sterile, tapered medical needles are sold at drugstores (you'll find them where the diabetic supplies are kept) and are easy on the skin. Do be sure that you have these on hand before attempting to pop any blemish.

The correct way to do an extraction is to start with the proper supplies. Along with the lancets, gather together your cleanser and exfoliator, a clean washcloth, some tissues, your witch hazel, and your Neosporin.

Once you have everything you need, wash your hands and begin:

- Be sure that you've cleansed and exfoliated the area first, because that layer of dead cells can hold an infection in and prevent the release of the clogged material.

- Soak the washcloth in hot water. Wring it out and hold it over the area of the pimple for about one minute. This softens the skin.

- Wrap your index fingers in tissues to cushion your nails. And be sure that your nails are short, since this is not safe to do with long ones!

- Start with blackheads, gently squeezing them with your wrapped nails.

- Do the whiteheads or cystic pimples next, but only if they're ready. Carefully pierce the center by pushing the lancet straight in and straight out. This provides the "canal" I talked about. Do *not* reuse lancets! Discard them after using.

- Gently squeeze with your wrapped fingers.

- Dab all of the extracted areas with witch hazel. If a spot is red and inflamed, apply a little Neosporin.

Here's a tip: If you are heavy-handed and tend to squeeze too hard, use Q-tips instead of tissue-wrapped fingers. You won't be able to press as intensely.

STEP 5: TREATMENT MASK

Look for something with minerals to calm any inflammation. If you've done a lot of extractions, a clay mask is a great choice because it will pull any remaining infection out of the pores and close them down.

Here are a few other at-home versions:

— *Honey mask:* Honey is a great hydrator, so it will attract water to your skin cells and then lock it in. Honey also has antimicrobial properties, so it's great for all skin types, especially the acne prone or dry.

Take a teaspoon of honey and massage it onto your clean skin. Leave the honey mask on for about ten minutes and then rinse with warm water. Your skin will feel so soft and smooth.

— *Brewer's-yeast mask:* This is great for oily skin, particularly for congestion or clogged pores. If you have combination skin, however, avoid the dry areas of your face.

Warm two teaspoons of water in the microwave in a small bowl. Add a packet of dry brewer's yeast to the warm water and mix it up. You'll want the mask to be about the same consistency or thickness of peanut butter; once it is, massage onto the skin. Leave it on for about ten minutes or until completely dry. You'll notice really clear skin and tight pores. But beware: this is pretty stinky!

Skin-telligence:

THE PIMPLE POLICE! If you have a pimple the day of a big event, don't pick it! In this case, it's better to wrap an ice cube in a thin cloth or paper towel and rest it on the blemish for a few minutes. The ice will reduce the inflammation and redness. Also, taking an aspirin, which has anti-inflammatory properties, will temporarily reduce the swelling.

— *Egg-white mask:* Egg whites are high in vitamin A and are effective for drying blemishes and for overall toning and tightening of the complexion. Suitable for all skin types, we even do a version of this mask at the clinic.

Separate one egg white into a bowl and stir slightly. With a brush or a cotton pad, apply the egg white onto your face. Allow it to dry, which should take about ten minutes, and then wash it off with warm water.

STEP 6: HYDRATE AND MOISTURIZE

Work in your serum all over your face and then finish with your favorite evening moisturizer, or try this:

— *Natural oils:* Olive and grapeseed oils can be effective moisturizers, although very simple. Just be careful if you're acne prone, as I believe they can possibly clog pores.

STEP 7: EYE TREATMENT

Grab your favorite eye cream, and dab it on. Don't forget to put it between your eyes, where the brow furrows; and across the bridge of your nose, where the skin is thinner and more prone to wrinkling.

Try the following for dark circles and puffy eyes:

— *Potato poultice:* Grab a cool potato from the fridge and chop it into very small pieces. Bind them in two pieces of cheesecloth, and place the poultices on your eyes for ten minutes. Or, simply use potato slices that have been soaked in cool water. Both methods help improve tired eyes.

— *Tea time:* Steep two bags of green tea in hot water, and allow the bags time to cool. Lie down and place one bag over each eye. The caffeine in the tea will help tighten the tissue, as well as reduce puffiness.

— *Spoon solution:* Place two spoons in the fridge or freezer for 15 to 30 minutes, and then lay them across your eyes for about 5 minutes. The cold metal will help de-puff and reduce tired circles. (I always do this when I travel!)

Extra Steps to Make It a More "Kate Somerville" Experience

- Get into your coziest robe and cushiest slippers.
- Light a fragrance-free soy or pure beeswax candle, since they don't give off any toxic smoke.
- Put on your favorite soothing music.
- Enjoy a glass of cool water with slices of cucumber or a squeeze of lemon juice.
- Turn off your phone's ringer.

Now that you've had a little you time, it's time for some more! In the next chapter, I give you a chart that tells you what ingredients and treatments work best for your skin type. It's almost like a "cheat sheet," and it's a helpful summary of all the treatments and ingredients you've learned about in the earlier chapters.

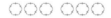

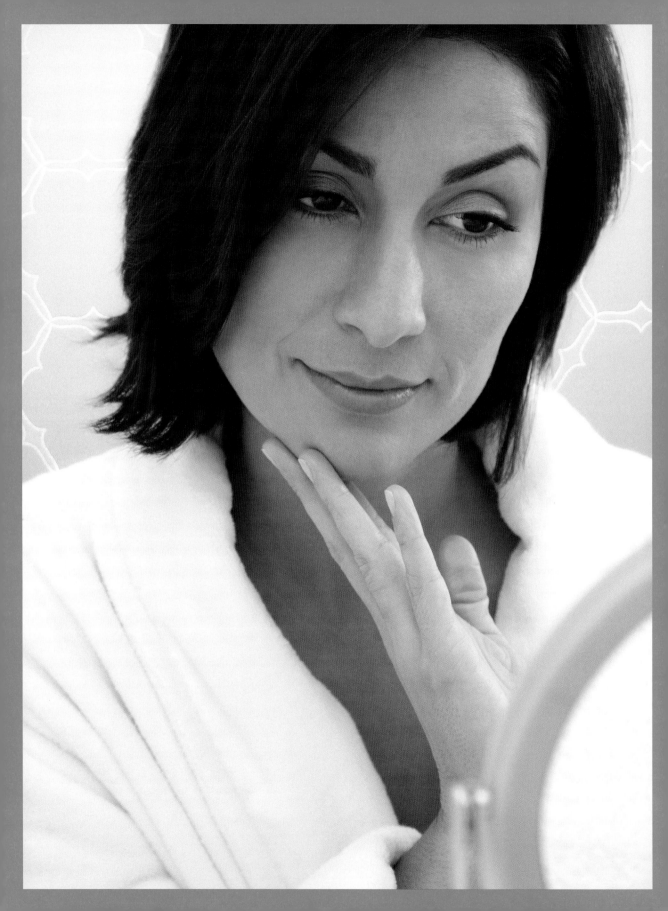

CHAPTER 9

Your Personal Skin Stategy

I realize that I've just given you a lot of information. So for those times when you need a refresher or a quick reference, here are my suggestions for your skin type, including ingredients, treatments, diet, and lifestyle. (**Note:** While I don't mention sunscreen or give dietary recommendations for every skin type in this chapter, everyone should use sunscreen and eat nutritious foods.)

SKIN TYPE: NORMAL

TREATMENTS

INGREDIENT AND DIET/LIFESTYLE RECOMMENDATIONS

- Regular facials, every six to eight weeks (these will help you stay on top of/prevent changes in your skin)
- In general, keep things simple: "If it isn't broken, don't fix it!"

- Cleansers: sulfate-free cleansers
- Exfoliators: fruit enzymes, glycolic acid
- Hydrators/moisturizers: emollients such as glycerin and hyaluronic acid
- Broad-spectrum sunscreen, chemical or physical
- Supplements: antioxidants including vitamins C and E

SKIN TYPE: DRY

TREATMENTS

INGREDIENT AND DIET/LIFESTYLE RECOMMENDATIONS

- Regular facials, every four weeks—be sure to choose hydrating or oxygen facials, such as my DermalQuench Oxygen Treatment
- Ultrasound facial treatments
- Dermaplaning
- Microcurrent

- Cleansers: gel or cream sulfate-free cleansers
- Exfoliators: fruit enzymes, glycolic acid
- Hydrators/moisturizers: glycerin, hyaluronic acid, ceramides, shea butter
- Diet: eat salmon and avocado; avoid caffeine
- Drink eight to ten glasses of purified water a day
- Take baths with colloidal oatmeal and immediately seal in moisture with lotion or natural oil
- Supplements: essential fatty acids

Dry skin is the result of dead skin cells— so be sure to exfoliate regularly if you fit into this category.

SKIN TYPE: SENSITIVE

TREATMENTS

- Red LED phototherapy
- Oxygen facials, every eight weeks—make sure to tell your facialist about ingredients and techniques that don't work for you, and facial massage is not recommended
- Avoid anything too aggressive or any facial treatment that could irritate your skin—and note that just because something says it's "natural," this doesn't mean it's good for sensitive skin

INGREDIENT AND DIET/LIFESTYLE RECOMMENDATIONS

- Cleansers: sulfate-free gel or cream cleansers
- Exfoliators: fruit enzymes, lactic acid (only if your skin can handle them)
- Hydrators/moisturizers: babassu oil, honey, essential fatty acids
- Calming agents: mineral masks, aloe, lavender, calendula, azulene, green tea, blue lotus
- Sunscreens with physical block: titanium dioxide or zinc
- Avoid products containing: alcohol, synthetic fragrance, colorants
- Diet: avoid spicy foods, caffeine, white sugar, white flour
- Pay attention to your body and how it responds to irritants like certain foods, laundry detergents, and perfumes

SKIN TYPE: OILY

TREATMENTS

- Regular facials, every three to six weeks based on level of congestion
- Red LED phototherapy (to regulate oil production)
- Laser Genesis series (if pores are also enlarged)

INGREDIENT AND DIET/LIFESTYLE RECOMMENDATIONS

- Cleansers: foaming cleansers, salicylic-acid cleansers
- Exfoliators: fruit enzymes, glycolic or lactic acids, round beads
- Hydrators/moisturizers: oil-free form-ulations with aloe vera, hyaluronic acid, HSC complex
- Ingredients that reduce oil: phytic acid, salicylic acid, witch hazel, tea-tree or peppermint oil, clay masks
- Avoid certain occlusives: mineral oil, petrolatum, coconut oil
- Diet: reduce saturated fats; drink eight to ten glasses of water a day
- Supplements: multivitamin with clean-sing herbs, vitamin A, zinc

SKIN TYPE: COMBINATION

TREATMENTS	INGREDIENT AND DIET/LIFESTYLE RECOMMENDATIONS
<ul><li>Regular facials, every four to six weeks</li><li>Laser Genesis series (to refine pores in oilier areas)</li><li>Ultrasound facial treatments</li></ul>	<ul><li>Cleansers: sulfate-free cleansers</li><li>Exfoliators: fruit enzymes; glycolic, salicylic, and lactic acids</li><li>Remember the ecosystem: use products for oily skin where you're oily, products for dry skin where you're dry, and products for acne where you're broken out</li><li>Balance ingredients: mineral masks, aloe vera, botanicals such as rosemary or fireweed (also known as Canadian willowherb)</li><li>Drink eight to ten glasses of water a day</li><li>Steam a few times a week to help hydrate and rebalance the skin</li></ul>

SKIN TYPE: ACNE

TREATMENTS	INGREDIENT AND DIET/LIFESTYLE RECOMMENDATIONS
<ul><li>Regular facials, every three to four weeks</li><li>LED phototherapy (alternating blue and red light)—be sure to look for a practitioner who will provide exfoliation before placing you under the lights, for increased efficacy</li></ul>	<ul><li>Cleansers: sulfate-free gel cleansers</li><li>Exfoliators: fruit enzymes, glycolic or lactic acids</li><li>Hydrators/moisturizers: oil-free formulations with aloe vera, hyaluronic acid</li><li>Ingredients that reduce oil/acne: phytic acid, salicylic acid, tea-tree oil, benzoyl peroxide, sulfur, clay masks, vitamin A</li><li>Avoid certain occlusives: mineral oil, petrolatum, coconut oil</li><li>Topical antibiotics if necessary: clindamycin, erythromycin</li><li>Diet: reduce saturated fats; avoid dairy, nonorganic meats, white sugar, and white flour; increase fiber; drink eight to ten glasses of water a day</li><li>Supplements: probiotics, vitamin A, zinc, cleansing herbs (burdock, dandelion)</li><li>Reduce stress, exercise</li></ul>

Please do not scrub too hard if you have blemishes! You can break them open and spread bacteria. Let the enzymes do the work.

SKIN TYPE: MATURE

TREATMENTS	INGREDIENT AND DIET/LIFESTYLE RECOMMENDATIONS
■ Regular facials, every six to eight weeks ■ Microcurrent ■ Ultrasound facial treatments ■ LED phototherapy (red and white series recommended) ■ Titan laser ■ Laser Genesis ■ Pearl laser ■ Pearl Fractional ■ Botox ■ Injectables	■ Cleansers: sulfate-free gel or cream cleansers ■ Exfoliators: fruit enzymes, glycolic acid (if skin is thin, instead opt for lactic acid) ■ Hydrators/moisturizers: hyaluronic acid, HSC complex, ceramides, shea butter ■ Serums: alpha-lipoic acid, vitamins A and C ■ Line reducers: peptides, neuropeptides ■ Diet: eat salmon, blueberries, olive oil, green tea, leafy greens ■ Supplements: essential fatty acids, calcium, magnesium, B complex, antioxidants

SKIN TYPE: MATURE AND ACNE

TREATMENTS	INGREDIENT AND DIET/LIFESTYLE RECOMMENDATIONS
■ Regular facials, every four weeks ■ Titan laser ■ Laser Genesis ■ Pearl laser ■ Pearl Fractional ■ Botox ■ Injectables	■ Cleansers: sulfate-free gel cleansers ■ Exfoliators: fruit enzymes, glycolic or lactic acids, round beads ■ Hydrators/moisturizers: oil-free formulations with aloe vera, hyaluronic acid ■ Ingredients that reduce oil/acne and increase cell turnover: phytic acid, salicylic acid, tea-tree oil, benzoyl peroxide, vitamin A ■ Avoid certain occlusives: mineral oil, petrolatum, coconut oil ■ Topical antibiotics if necessary: clindamycin, erythromycin ■ Diet: reduce saturated fats; avoid dairy, nonorganic meats, white sugar, and white flour; increase fiber; drink eight to ten glasses of water a day ■ Supplements: probiotics, vitamin A, zinc, cleansing herbs (burdock, dandelion) ■ Reduce stress, exercise

SKIN TYPE: HYPERPIGMENTED

TREATMENTS

- IPL treatments (series of three to six); however, if you suspect that your hyper-pigmentation is melasma, avoid IPL (see the note about this treatment under Hyper-pigmented/Melasma below)
- Dermaplaning
- Ultrasound facial treatments (with use of brightening agents)
- Red LED phototherapy
- Cosmelan
- TCA peel (if pigmentation is very deep and stubborn)

INGREDIENT AND DIET/LIFESTYLE RECOMMENDATIONS

- Cleansers: containing natural brighteners
- Exfoliators: fruit enzymes, glycolic and lactic acids
- Natural brighteners: phytic acid, kojic acid, licorice extract, vitamins A and C
- Hydroquinone: use sparingly and with caution
- Sun protection: always wear sunblock (physical or chemical); wear a hat and sunglasses when outdoors
- Supplements: antioxidants and cleansing herbs, as well as those that boost internal SPF, such as pomegranate and green tea

SKIN TYPE: HYPERPIGMENTED/MELASMA

TREATMENTS

- Dermaplaning
- Ultrasound facial treatments (with use of brightening agents)
- Red LED phototherapy
- Cosmelan
- TCA peel (if pigmentation is very deep and stubborn)
- Avoid IPL—this is not recommended for melasma because it can contribute to more pigment production

INGREDIENT AND DIET/LIFESTYLE RECOMMENDATIONS

- Cleansers: containing natural brighteners
- Exfoliators: fruit enzymes, glycolic and lactic acids
- Natural brighteners: phytic acid, kojic acid, licorice extract, vitamins A and C
- Hydroquinone: use sparingly and with caution
- Sun protection: avoid long exposure to sun; always wear sunscreen and a hat
- Avoid intense heat: dry saunas can exacerbate melasma/pigmentation
- Diet: avoid dairy and nonorganic meats
- Supplements: antioxidants and cleansing herbs, as well as those that boost internal SPF, such as pomegranate and green tea
- Birth control pills: discuss low-estrogen pills and alternatives with your health-care professional

SKIN TYPE: SCARRED

TREATMENTS

- Titan laser (can help stimulate collagen where there are depression marks)
- Pearl Fractional
- Injectables
- LED phototherapy (red and white series recommended)

INGREDIENT AND DIET/LIFESTYLE RECOMMENDATIONS

- Cleansers: sulfate-free cleansers
- Exfoliators: fruit enzymes, glycolic and lactic acids
- Hydrators/moisturizers: hyaluronic acid, ceramides, shea butter, avocado oil
- Brighteners: vitamins A and C, kojic acid, licorice extract
- Collagen builders: peptides
- Diet: oily fish, walnuts, cranberries
- Supplements: essential fatty acids, antioxidants

SKIN TYPE: ROSACEA

TREATMENTS

- Laser Genesis
- IPL
- Red LED phototherapy
- Avoid microcurrent, acid peels, and dermaplaning

INGREDIENT AND DIET/LIFESTYLE RECOMMENDATIONS

- Cleansers: sulfate-free gel or cream cleansers
- Exfoliators: fruit enzymes (avoid acids, beads, and scrubbing)
- Hydrators/moisturizers: babassu oil, essential fatty acids
- Calming agents: mineral masks, aloe, lavender, calendula, azulene, green tea, blue lotus
- Sunscreens with physical block: titanium dioxide or zinc
- Avoid products containing alcohol, synthetic fragrance, and colorants
- Diet: avoid trigger foods such as caffeine, white sugar, white flour, alcohol, spicy foods
- Avoid steam rooms and dry saunas

I've suffered from eczema all my life. It's a challenging skin condition that takes a lot of time and effort to get under control. My first word of advice is: You must go see your dermatologist. Ask him or her for the prescription Clobetasol 0.05% cream.

Note that Clobetasol is a high-powered corticosteroid, so you'll apply it on the affected area three times a day for only five days. You do not want to overuse this cream—it can thin the skin permanently! When applying any medication, make sure you really massage it into the affected area. The medication needs to be "pushed" into the skin to be truly effective.

I use this corticosteroid cream sparingly— that is, only to control inflammation and get the eczema into remission. Unfortunately, for most people eczema is a condition that rarely goes away completely, and it's something we who suffer from it have to deal with throughout our lives.

The next key to the puzzle is this: Get into a lukewarm (not hot) bath for at least 20 minutes a day. This allows the water to absorb into, and soothe, the skin. It's important that you not use any type of soaps or detergents on your body or on the affected areas. When getting out of the bath, pat dry—*do not* rub or towel off completely, as this can aggravate the skin. Immediately apply Curél original lotion, which seals in the moisture and allows skin to recover. Of course, if you have eczema on your hands, Curél must be reapplied every time you wash them.

Within two weeks, your skin should start feeling much better. The key is to use the medication infrequently, reserving usage for when the eczema is intense. Again, use the Clobetasol three times daily for five days, and only in the spot where you feel that tingle. Additionally, try not to wear wool or itchy materials—only cottons and soft fabrics should be worn during flare-ups.

I've personally kept my eczema in check, in almost complete remission, as a result of following this protocol. It's been a lifelong battle, but I finally have it under control . . . and you can, too!

SKIN TYPE: ECZEMA

TREATMENTS

- LED phototherapy (red and white series recommended)
- Ultrasound facial treatments
- Avoid microcurrent and most lasers

INGREDIENT AND DIET/LIFESTYLE RECOMMENDATIONS

- Cleansers: sulfate-free cleansers
- Exfoliators: fruit enzymes
- Hydrators/moisturizers: gamma-linolenic acid (borage oil), hyaluronic acid, avocado oil, or my own Goat Milk Body Lotion
- Topical steroids: cortisone cream (used sparingly and only for severe outbreaks)
- Avoid products containing alcohol, synthetic fragrance, and colorants
- Diet: avoid spicy foods, caffeine, white sugar, white flour, alcohol, carbonation, wheat
- Supplements: omega-3 essential fatty acids, antioxidants, B complex, zinc
- Take baths with colloidal oatmeal; seal in moisture with Goat Milk Body Lotion or natural oil
- Pay attention to your body and how it responds to your environment and foods
- Keep bedding clean to reduce irritation associated with dust mites

I hope that this chapter will give you some specific guidance regarding your particular skin condition, and help you summarize a personal strategy.

Now that we've discovered what works for all skin types, let's see all of this in action. Bring on the skin transformations!

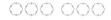

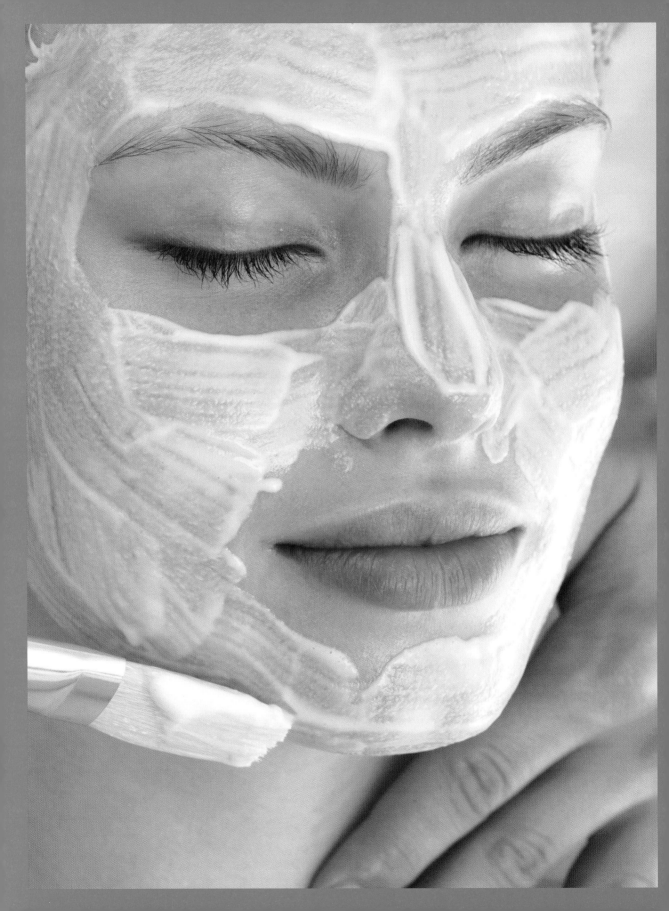

PART III

Complexion Transformation!

10 Weeks to Complexion Perfection!

In the first two parts of *Complexion Perfection!* you learned so much about the skin, about what makes it tick, and how to change what you don't like. Now you're going to see what I've been talking about—

in action. Skin makeovers! This is what I love to do,

and this is what I do best.

My responsibilities within my company are many. There's a lot of travel, personal appearances, media interviews, lectures, luncheons, trade shows—you name it. But transforming skin is what gives me my mojo, and it's why I do what I do. I'm inspired by the pure potential in someone's skin, and I love a challenge.

Life places its stamp upon your face, and that stamp may detract from the beauty of your true self. When you have severe acne, for instance, it's hard to let your spirit shine. Having a skin issue can be like wearing a mask all the time: the face that the world sees simply isn't *you*.

In this book, it was important for me to be able to show you what can be done with skin and just how responsive it can be. So as I was writing, I posed this question around the office, to friends of friends, and to neighbors of colleagues: "Who's up for a skin transformation?" Needless to say, my phone was ringing off the hook! The volunteers are from all walks of life, each with his or her own unique skin challenges. We have 13 women and 2 men, and their ages range from 19 to 71. The one thing all of these clients did have in common was that they weren't satisfied with the present state of their skin, and they couldn't figure out how to fix it.

Enter my team and me. First, Melissa (my registered nurse-practitioner) and I met with each client for a comprehensive skin evaluation. We got to know a little bit about each one of them personally, along with their individual skin struggles. We needed to do this so that we could best assess all factors contributing to the state of their complexions.

After the evaluations, Melissa and I came up with a treatment program for each client that included facial treatments, products, and diet/lifestyle suggestions. Then we took the "before" shots with completely clean skin. While the women may have had on just a touch of lip gloss and mascara to make them feel a bit more comfortable, their complexions were left naked and untouched.

Then we got to work: my team and I spent ten weeks transforming the skin of our volunteers. We only had ten weeks! The clients did their homework, and we did ours. Most of the men and women came in at least twice a week, and they stuck to their product regimens at home. (They also took home my product line, which you can learn more about in the My Products section at the end of the book.)

The photos you're about to see are *not* retouched, and the lighting is the same throughout; in other words, these are the real-deal results. Keep in mind that for most clients with serious concerns, my clinicians and I spend anywhere from six months to a year working on their skin. So just imagine how dramatic the results in this part of the book would be with a little more time! But what was most important to me was that you see that you don't have to go under the knife to take years off of your face, take damaging prescription drugs to get rid of embarrassing acne, or walk down the aisle with a mask of makeup to cover up stubborn pigment.

In describing what we did for each client, I haven't gone into all of the "whys," because the treatments and products have been fully laid out in preceding chapters. So if you're wondering why someone had Titan or used an oil-free moisturizer, flip back to the previous chapters and you'll understand.

Thanks to my team at the clinic and to the volunteers' desire and commitment, we witnessed powerful changes in skin that not only transformed faces, but also changed lives. The pictures of the following 15 people are almost as powerful as are their stories.

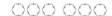

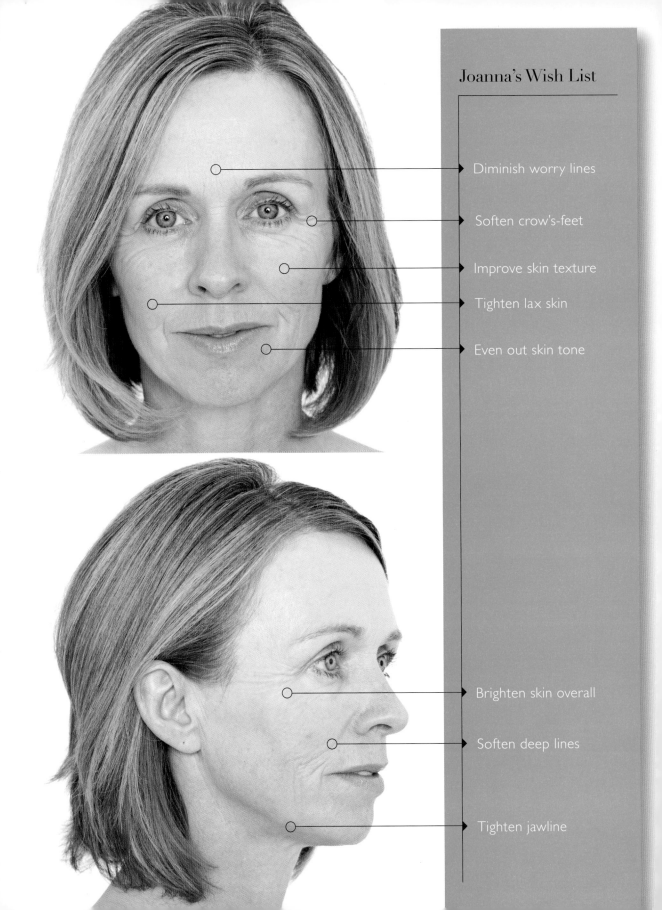

Joanna's Wish List

Diminish worry lines

Soften crow's-feet

Improve skin texture

Tighten lax skin

Even out skin tone

Brighten skin overall

Soften deep lines

Tighten jawline

Anti-aging

Joanna travels back and forth between her homes in England and California. She's an entrepreneur who runs a luxury water-filtration business, and she's the mother of four. Two of those children are twins, who were four months old at the time we took her "before" picture. "I have a very blessed life, but I do put a lot of energy into my husband and my kids. I'm a hands-on, busy mom," she said. "I go at 100 miles an hour."

Growing up in England, Joanna was outdoorsy, riding horses every day out in harsh, cold weather. She was lucky in that she missed the "acne years" and has always had clear skin. But she admitted, "I had no clue how to take care of my skin, and I think it got old too quickly. I'm not ready to look this age." She hadn't been happy with a photograph of herself for at least five years, which I think is something many people can identify with. "I don't mind the lines," she told me, "because they give character to the face. It's the drooping and sagging I want to get rid of."

Joanna has been good about getting regular facials, which she said left her skin feeling clean, but she'd been hoping to see herself looking ten years younger and hadn't seen any lasting changes. A friend of hers is a longtime client of mine, and she suggested that Joanna would be a good candidate for one of our makeovers.

My Analysis

The texture of Joanna's skin was fabulous, and there wasn't a lot we needed to do. Her problems were mostly skin laxity and dryness.

I decided that we could achieve results for Joanna mainly with lasers and Botox (after first making sure that she'd finished breast-feeding her twins). I told her that we could do injectables as well, if she was open to that, but she said that she'd prefer to stick with the other treatments and see how far that took her.

PRODUCTS

Step 1: Cleanse

■ Gentle Daily Wash morning and night

Step 2: Exfoliate

■ ExfoliKate Intensive Exfoliating Treatment twice a week

■ Micro Glycolic Polisher once a week as a serum left overnight

Step 3: Treat

■ Quench Hydrating Serum morning and night

Step 4: Moisturize

■ Deep Tissue Repair and Line Release Under Eye Repair Cream morning and night

Step 5: Protect

■ Protect SPF 30 Sunscreen

- Laser Genesis®
- Titan®
- Pearl® (two treatments)

- Botox®
- Omnilux™ white and red LED lights

DIET AND LIFESTYLE RECOMMENDATIONS

- Add flaxseed oil to her diet to help with skin dryness

- Take baths rather than showers, and apply moisturizer immediately to seal in the water

- Take my Total Vitamin Anti-Aging Supplement

The Results

After Joanna had her first Pearl treatment, she was trying to decide if she needed another when her 13-year-old son said, "Do it, Mommy. It's really working." And when Joanna's mother visited from England, she was so impressed by her daughter's dramatic results that she came in for a facial treatment, too.

Joanna's skin has taken on a beautiful, healthy sheen. Although she opted for no injectable fillers, strategically placed Botox has lessened some of the lines around her eyes and mouth. She's now a total convert, vowing to keep up with the Botox. We worked our magic with the lasers and LED lights, and she looks absolutely amazing. "Feeling better about my skin has really permeated my whole life," she shared. "I don't even mind having photos taken anymore." I can't say that I blame her, since in the "after" photos, her skin is just about glowing off of the page!

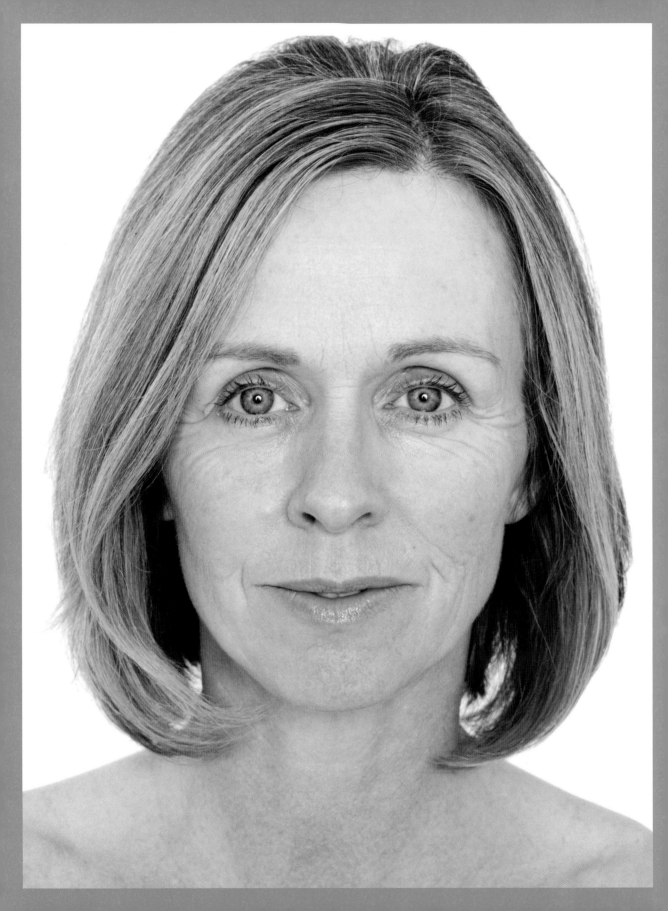

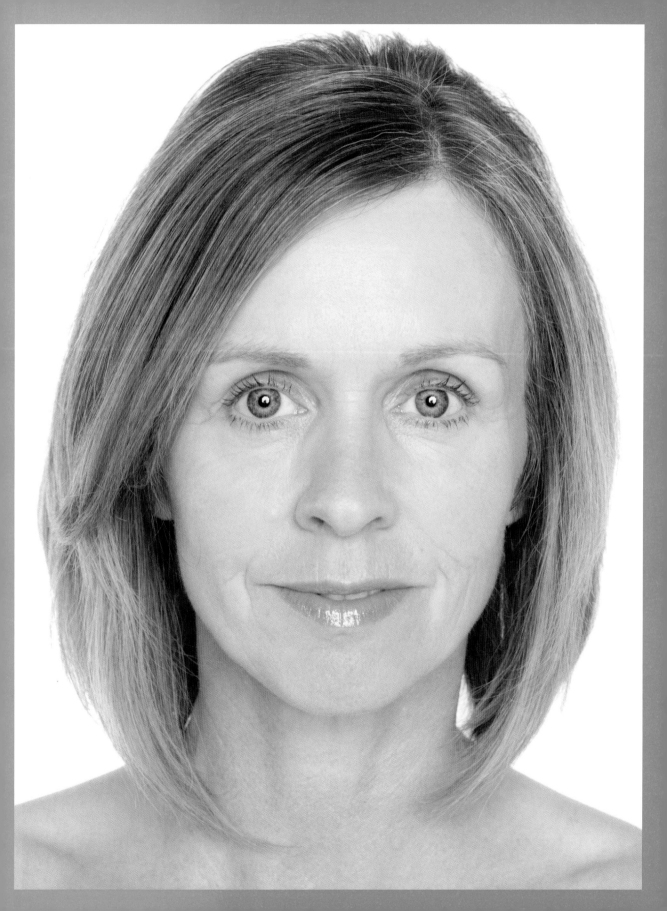

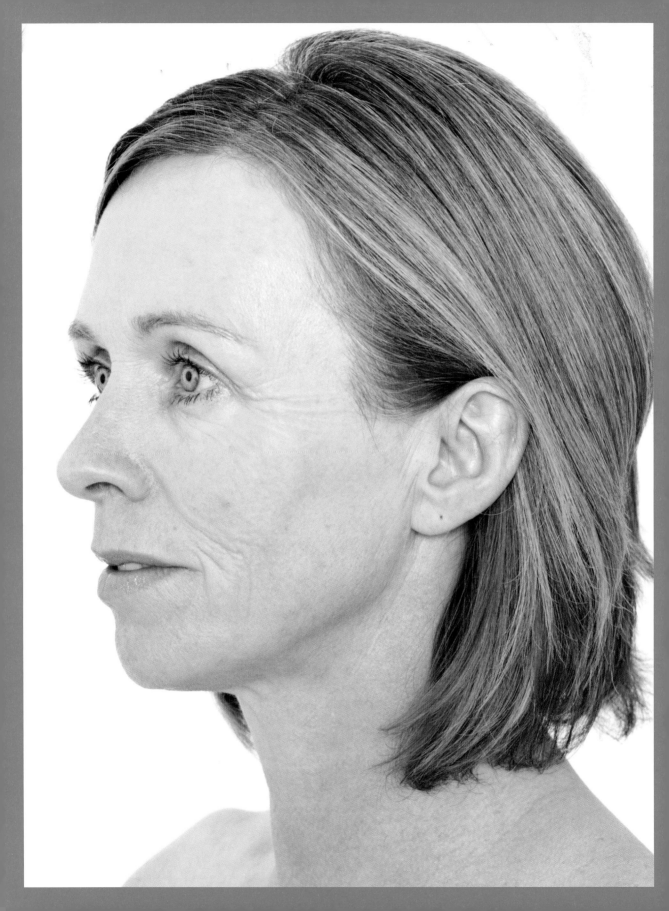

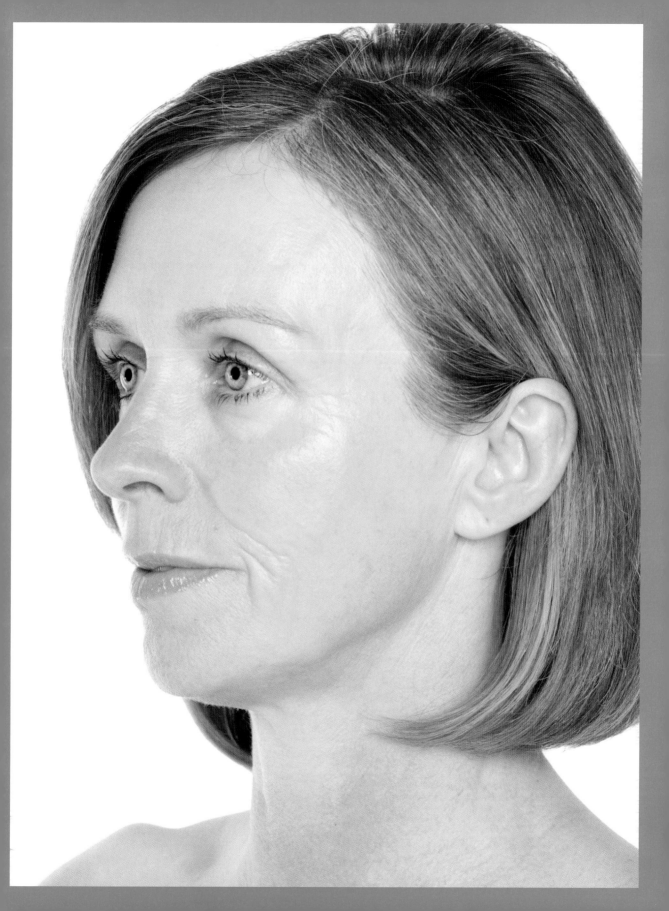

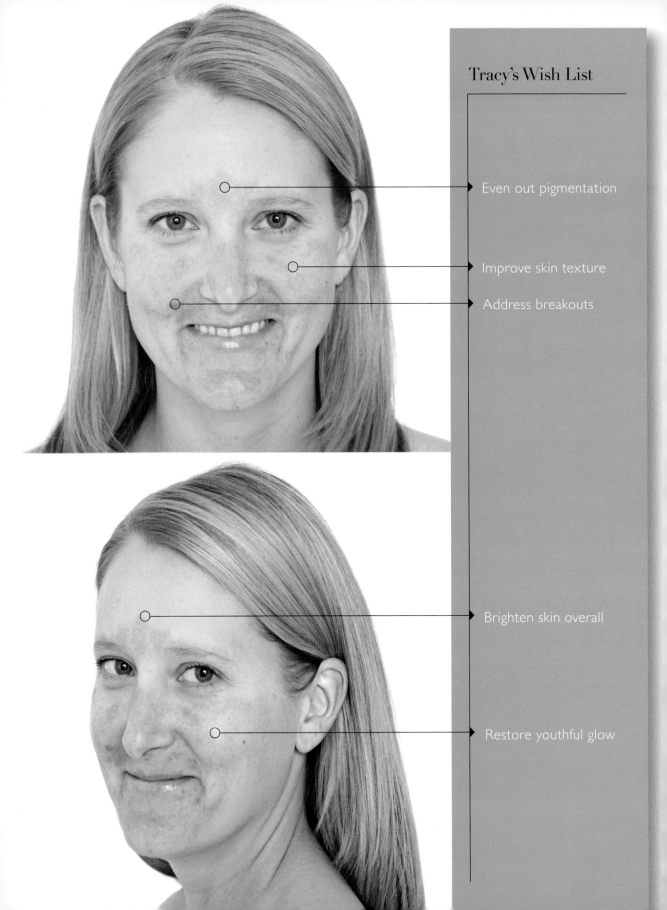

Tracy's Wish List

Even out pigmentation

Improve skin texture

Address breakouts

Brighten skin overall

Restore youthful glow

Melasma (discoloration), breakouts

Tracy is an ER nurse at Cedars-Sinai Medical Center in Los Angeles. She had acne as a teenager and tried everything to clear it up.

Because she got frustrated and also came from a family where people didn't spend time thinking about their skin, she fell into a habit of neglecting hers. Even though she's very active outdoors, she admitted to not even wearing sunscreen. "I've never had anyone sit me down and tell me what I should be doing and using," she confessed. Did she ever come to the right place!

Her melasma—discoloration—had come up in the last few years. Although she'd been aware of it, it was only when she moved to L.A. that she became self-conscious. "Everyone cares what they look like here," Tracy said. "I've had at least ten people I don't even know come up to me at work to comment on my skin and offer names of doctors or remedies!" While she knows that these people are only trying to be helpful, the attention has made her feel bad about herself.

Tracy came to the clinic several months prior to getting married at an eco-resort, and I promised her a fresh face for the occasion. Clear and natural is her ideal vision for her skin. As she told me, "I want to be able to just go out without wearing makeup and feel confident about how I look."

My Analysis

Tracy's discoloration was clearly melasma: it was on her face, cheeks, and forehead in an obvious symmetrical pattern characteristic of the condition. While she did have a minor breakout of acne, my concern was to get rid of this irregular coloring and restore healthy, evenly pigmented skin. I knew that my team could do it, but I also knew that it wouldn't be easy, since melasma is stubborn. My plan was to treat it down to the "root" cell so that it wouldn't continue to influence the healthy cells. We needed to turn over the cells fast; in this way, we could control what was happening deep down.

Tracy's acne was sporadic, and I decided it could be treated topically, with a simple product regimen. Yet for this young woman, I stressed compliance. She *had* to follow instructions, or she wouldn't get the results she wanted.

PRODUCTS

Step 1: Cleanse

- Gentle Daily Wash morning and night

Step 2: Exfoliate

- ExfoliKate Intensive Exfoliating Treatment twice a week

- Micro Glycolic Polisher once a week as a serum

Step 3: Treat

- Refrigerator Cream (which is something we custom-blend in the clinic and is a combination of Retin-A, hydroquinone, and a little bit of cortisone), to use only on the pigmented areas. Since this is a medication, I made sure that Tracy knew it was important to use the full dose every night.

- Clearing Mask on pimples overnight

Step 4: Moisturize

- Oil Free Moisturizer for day

- Nourish Daily Moisture for night

Step 5: Protect

- Protect SPF 30 Sunscreen

CLINIC TREATMENTS

- Laser Genesis®
- DermaLucent™ red light
- Pearl®
- Cosmelan®

DIET AND LIFESTYLE RECOMMENDATION

- Take my Total Vitamin Anti-Aging Supplement

The Results

"My results are incredible!" Tracy concluded. "The melasma is completely gone just about everywhere, and where it was really bad, it's faded to where it's hardly noticeable." She told me that jaws drop when people see her (mine certainly did at her final result!). All of those "helpful" comments she used to get have stopped—instead, people are now coming up to her and complimenting her on how beautiful her skin looks and asking her what she's doing. "It's been a total reverse effect," she told me. Her fiancé was supportive throughout the process, even though he thought she was just fine as she was. However, now Tracy can go forward with her wedding knowing that she has the fresh, radiant skin she wanted. And the bonus is that these days, she never leaves the house without sunscreen.

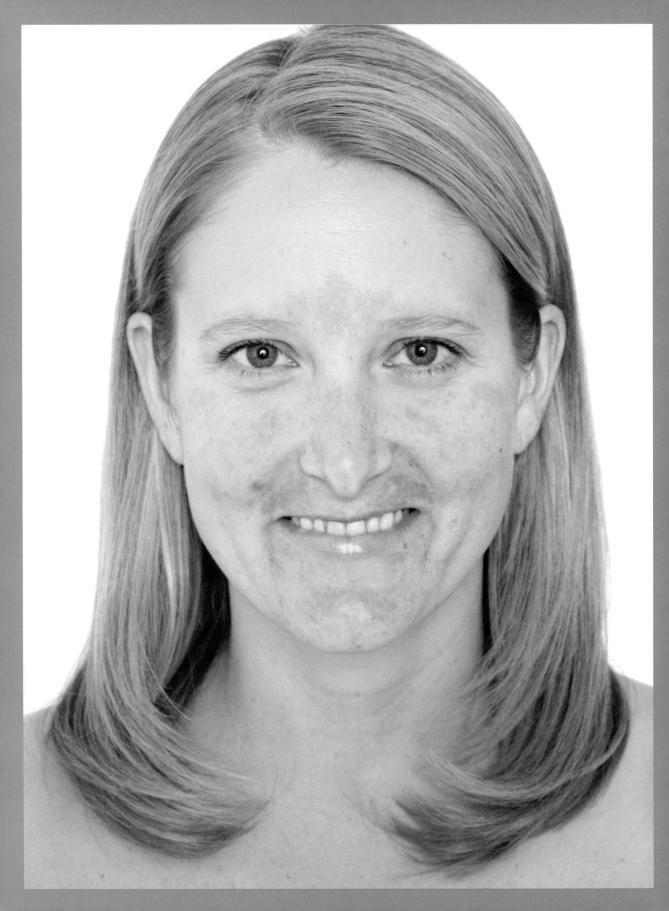

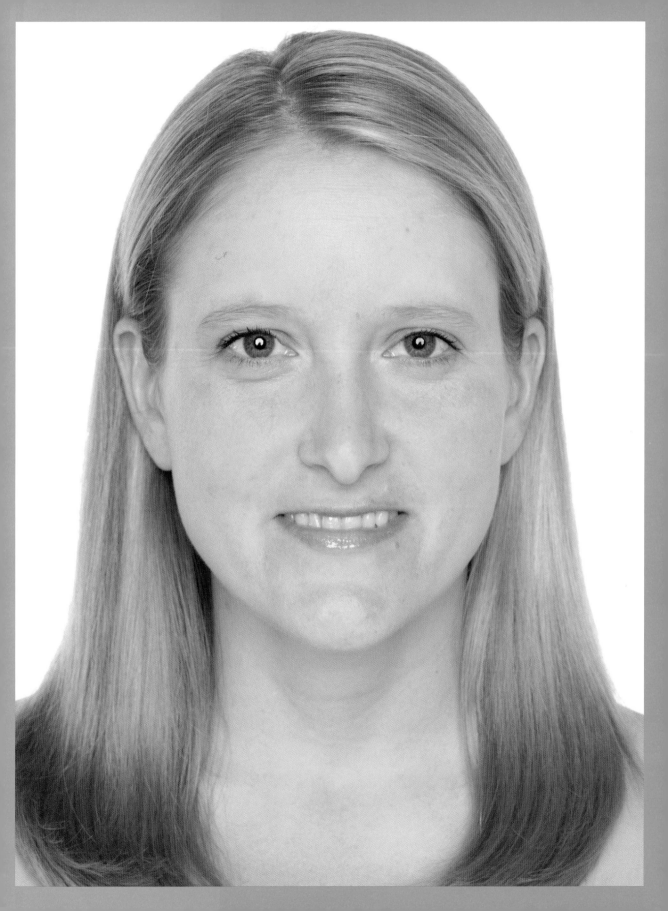

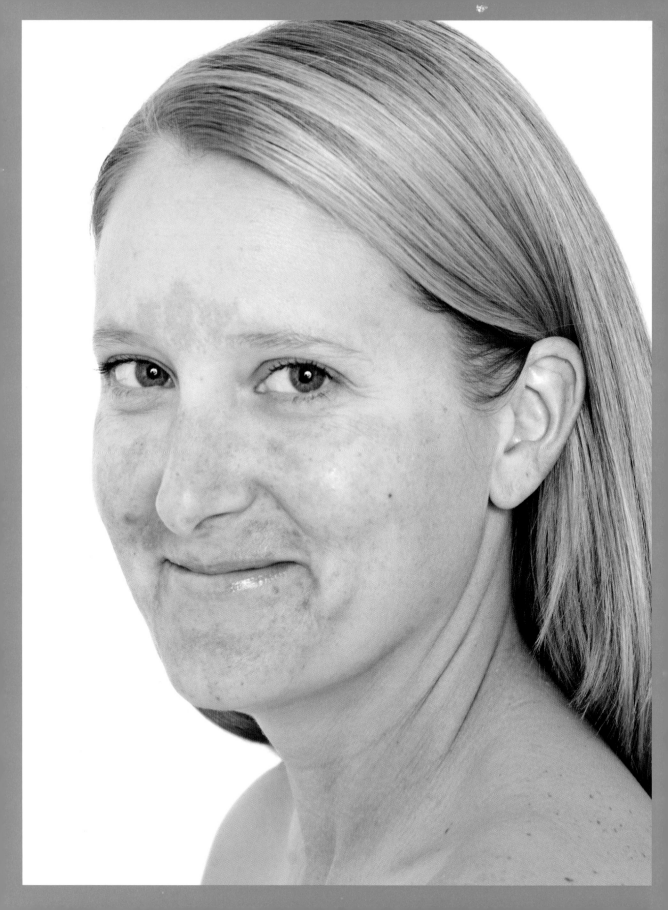

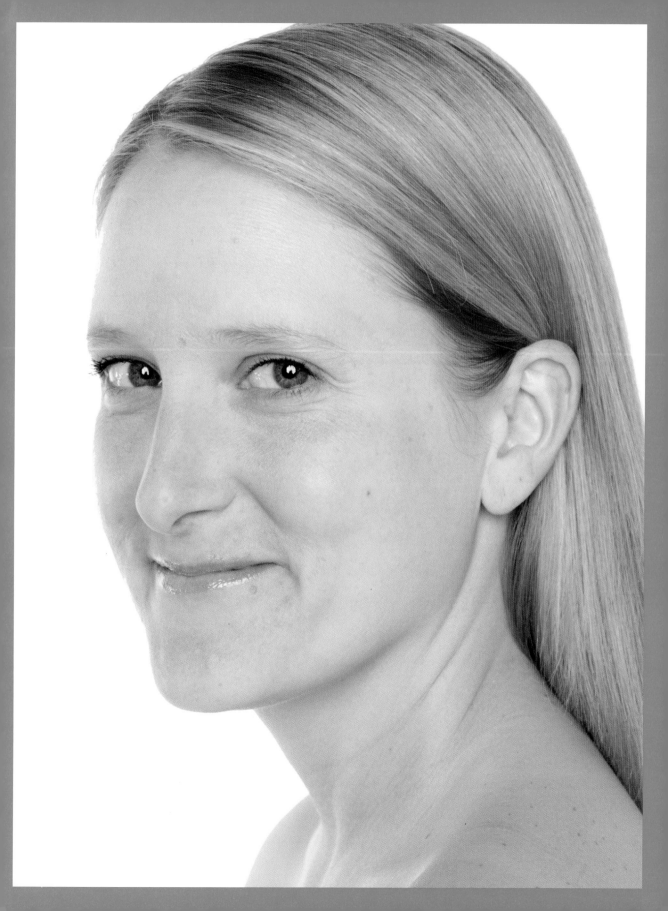

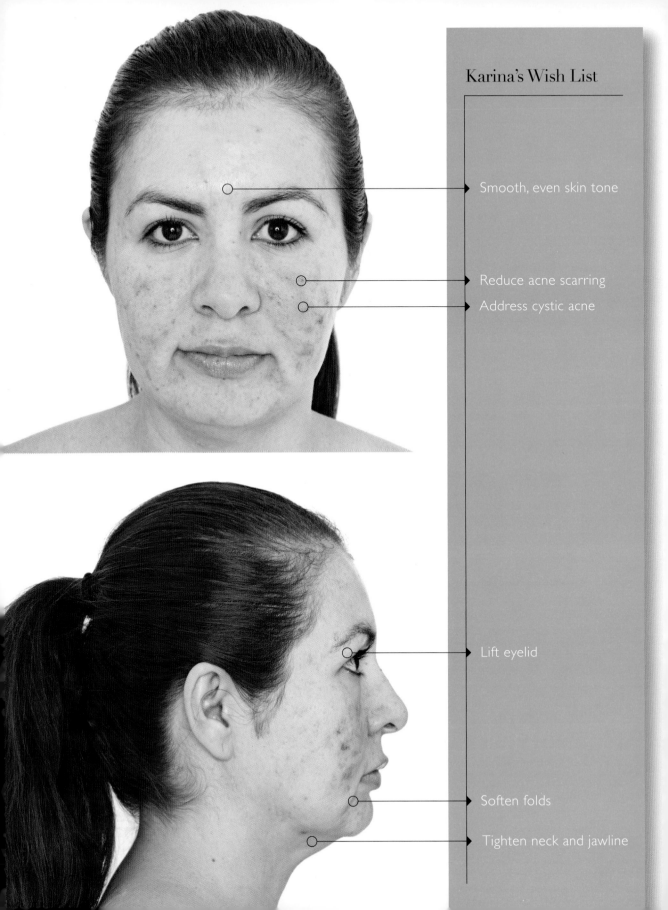

Karina's Wish List

Smooth, even skin tone

Reduce acne scarring

Address cystic acne

Lift eyelid

Soften folds

Tighten neck and jawline

Anti-aging, acne

"I feel self-conscious because sometimes my acne will look like a rash," Karina said. "My face can also look red and puffy, and I've actually had people ask me if I was hit in the face." She does fashion consulting and technical design, which means that she moves in a world where physical appearance matters. She wanted to get to the point where she didn't have to worry about how she looked if she had an event. "I've actually postponed meetings with new clients because they might make assumptions about me," she confessed. "I'll put off something really important and try to get my skin to look just a little better." I really felt for her.

Karina's acne started when she was young, but she always seemed to manage it, getting at least temporary results from visits to the dermatologist. Recently, though, she had some medical issues and told me, "Even washing your face isn't a priority when you're sick, so I wasn't taking care of myself." On top of that, she was required to take hormones, and the medication did a number on her complexion. Now that she feels healthier, she wants to get her skin in shape.

Like many of the other makeover candidates, this woman also dreams about not having to pile on makeup to get out the door: "Even if I'm only taking my son to school, I put on makeup because I don't want to be embarrassed. I'd like to be able to just put on some sunblock or something light and go out."

My Analysis

Karina's acne was a pretty extreme case, and it was coupled with acne scarring. Her condition had improved a bit since she'd gone off hormone therapy, but cystic acne and discoloration from past breakouts still existed. She also needed to have the texture smoothed out and some tightening around her jawline. I wanted to make her feel good about herself and put a smile on her face again.

PRODUCTS

Step 1: Cleanse

- Detox Daily Cleanser morning and night

- Clarifying Treatment Toner once a day, morning or night

Step 2: Exfoliate

- ExfoliKate Intensive Exfoliating Treatment twice a week

- Clearing Mask at night, only where she's broken out

Step 3: Treat

- Anti Bac Clearing Lotion once a day, in the morning, on acne

Step 4: Moisturize

- Oil Free Moisturizer morning and night

Step 5: Protect

- Protect SPF 30 Sunscreen

- Two Omnilux™ LED anti-acne series (blue/red light)
- Laser Genesis®
- Titan®
- Pearl®

- Botox®
- Restylane®
- Radiesse®
- Juvéderm®

DIET AND LIFESTYLE RECOMMENDATION

- Take my Total Vitamin Clear Skin Supplement

The Results

Karina had jaw-dropping (and lifting!) results. In fact, she now refers to her "old face" and her "new face." After 20 years of going to dermatologists and taking harsh medications, she finally saw some relief from her acne and old scars. She's a big fan of the Pearl, seeing a huge change in her texture and tone from it.

"I'm absolutely going to continue treatments at the clinic once or twice a month," Karina pledged. After experiencing the transformation this makeover has made in her life, treatments are no longer an option for her; they're a necessity.

You could just see the change in Karina's entire face: she had a light in her eyes, which was my goal. She said that her entire personality at work and even home changed in that she now sets up meetings instead of avoiding them. Her son is so happy that it doesn't take two hours for her to get ready before she takes him to school anymore. He joins us in being incredibly proud of how beautiful she looks.

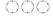

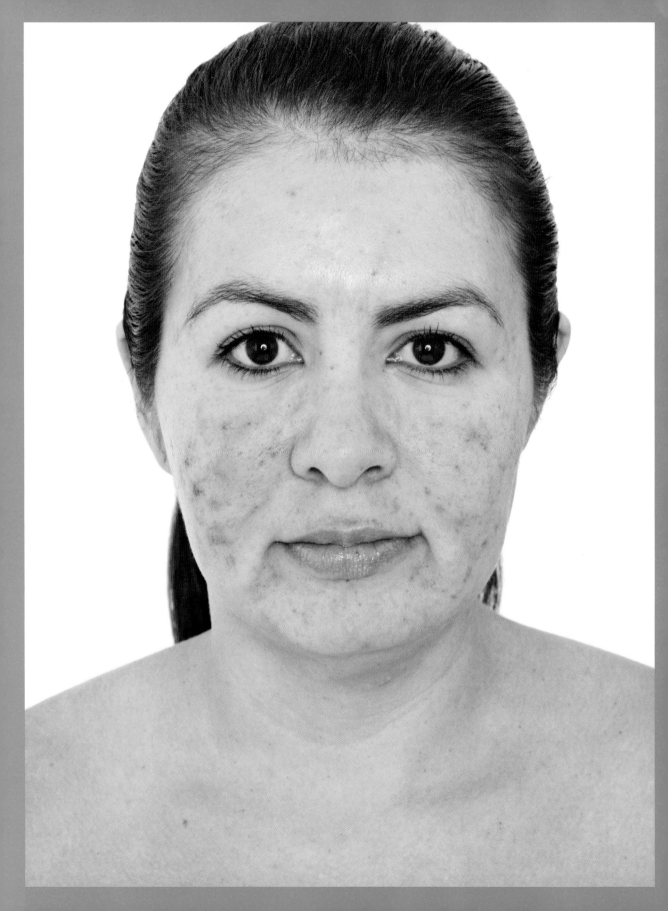

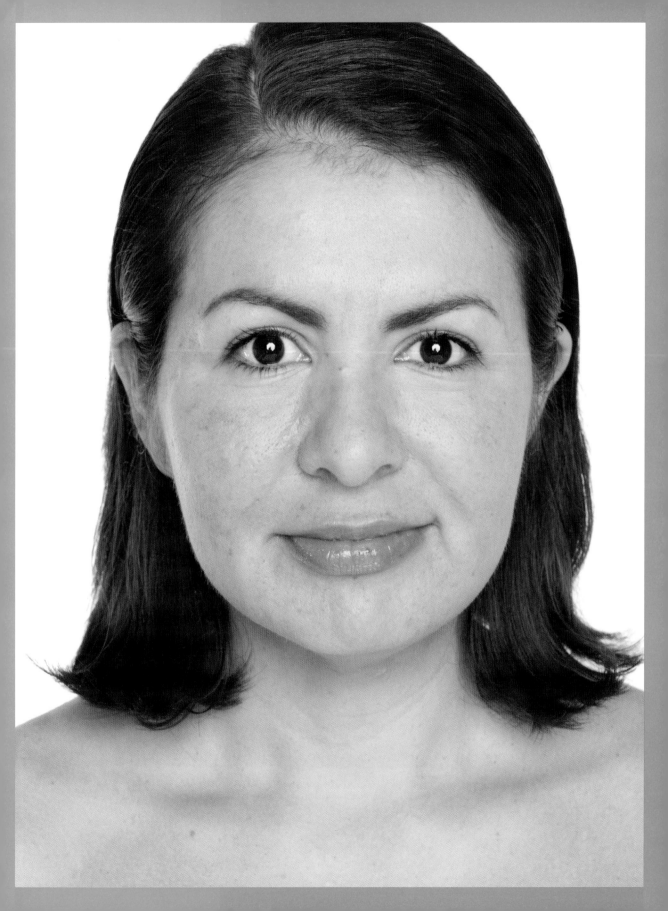

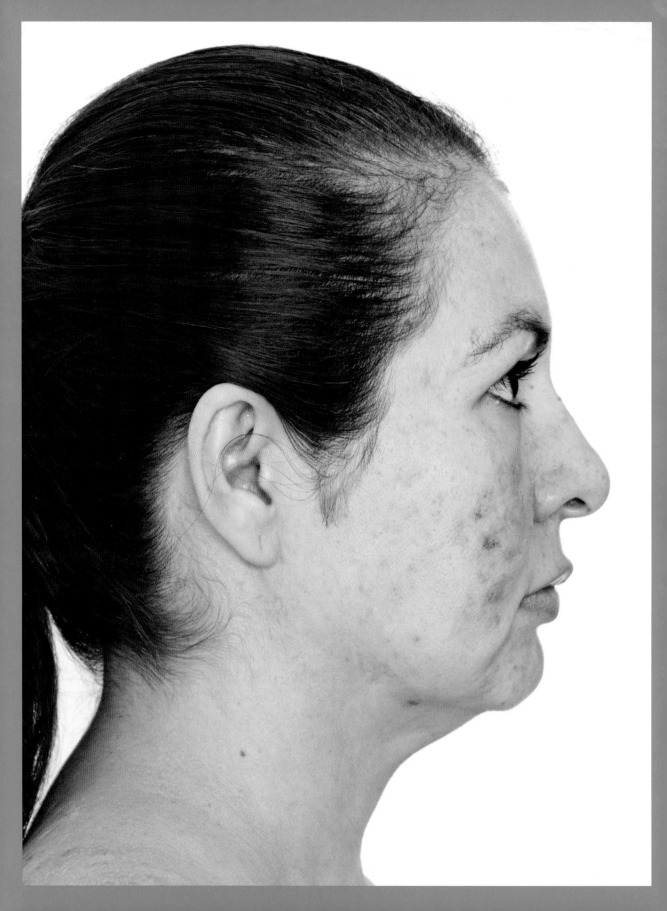

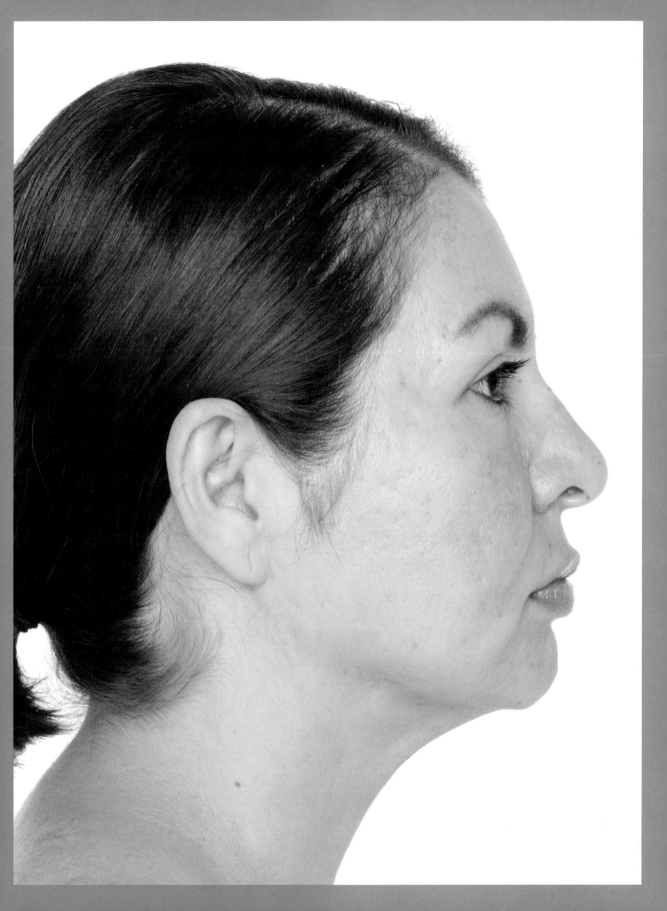

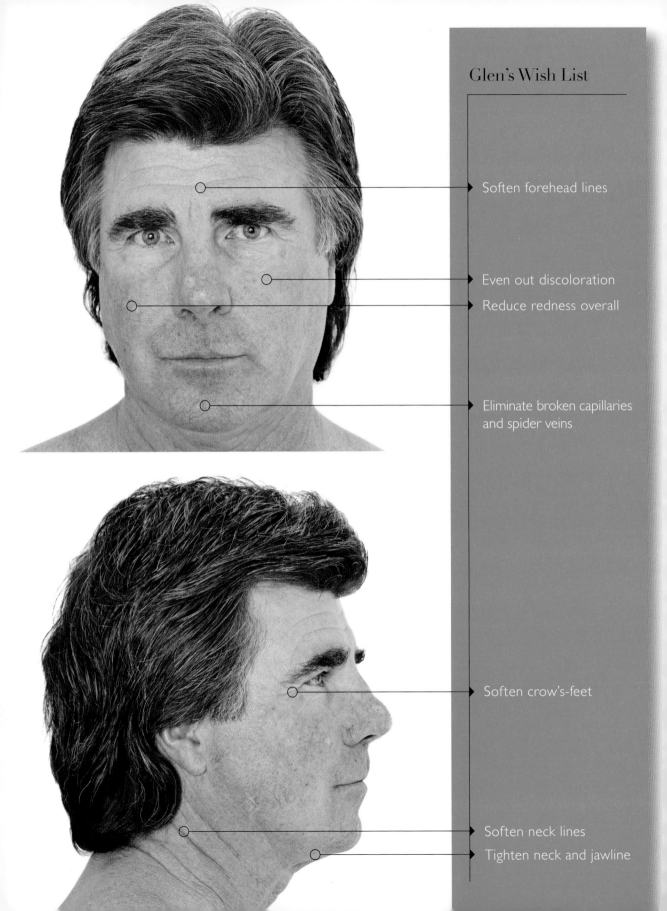

Glen's Wish List

Soften forehead lines

Even out discoloration

Reduce redness overall

Eliminate broken capillaries and spider veins

Soften crow's-feet

Soften neck lines

Tighten neck and jawline

Redness, anti-aging

Glen is a great guy who works in the apparel industry, and he's also the father of one of my colleagues. Hailing from Southern California, he's been a lifetime surfer and plays golf regularly. "I've always been in the sun," he said. "I used to get tan, but as I've gotten older, my skin has gotten redder." He does use sunscreen, but he doesn't like the feeling of most of them or the fact that they tend to clog his pores.

Apart from the redness, Glen mentioned that his skin is extremely dry after he washes and shaves his face in the morning. But he's remarkably unlined for his age, which he attributes to a combination of good genes (his mother is alive and well at 101!) and a generally healthy lifestyle: he gave up sugar three years ago, eats a lot of fish and chicken along with the occasional burger, and exercises regularly.

"I've noticed that I don't look as old as my friends do," Glen says. "I'm in the fashion business, so it's good to look younger than I am." He isn't too self-conscious about his skin, but he does get tired of people asking him if he "just got back from skiing" or "went to the beach." He's interested to see the results, joking, "Perhaps I'll look like I did in my 30s!"

My Analysis

Glen was one of the lucky ones who didn't have a lot of aging signs, but his skin was noticeably red, and he had visible veins—some small, and some larger than others—mostly around his nose, on the sides of his face, and on his chin. He needed laser vascular therapy and light treatments to calm the redness. I also switched him to my own sunscreen, which is not waxy or clogging.

PRODUCTS

Step 1: Cleanse

- Gentle Daily Wash in the morning

Step 2: Exfoliate

- ExfoliKate Intensive Exfoliating Treatment twice a week

Step 3: Treat

- Quench Hydrating Face Serum morning and night

Step 4: Moisturize

- Oil Free Moisturizer morning and night

Step 5: Protect

- Protect SPF 55 Serum Sunscreen

- CoolGlide Vascular Therapy
- IPL
- Laser Genesis®
- Omnilux™ white and red LED lights

The Results

The day before we took our "after" photos, somebody guessed Glen's age as 47! So he didn't quite make it back to his 30s, but he was very pleased anyway. That was not the only compliment he's received: co-workers and friends have noticed the improvement in his skin, and his wife is especially appreciative.

The redness that Glen's lived with for years subsided a lot, and his vascular problems were an easy fix. As he noted, "It was amazing to see how the capillaries disappeared immediately." But he was just as pleased with "the comfort factor" as he was with his appearance. "My face doesn't feel dry and flaky in the morning anymore," he told me. "It's really soft now. Feel?" He's become a believer in using moisturizer and intends to keep up a regimen of regular product use and treatments. I love it when the men convert!

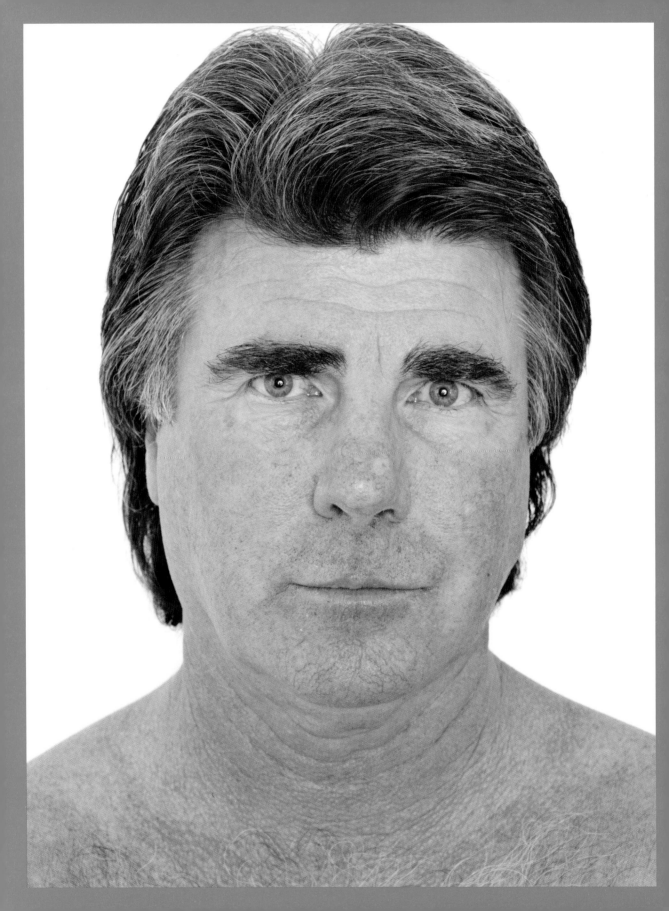

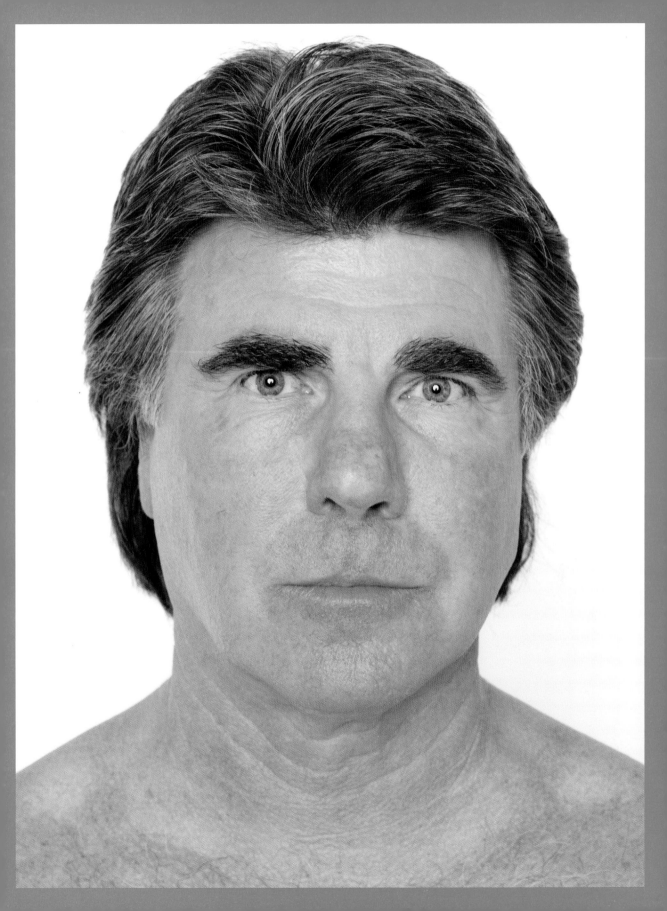

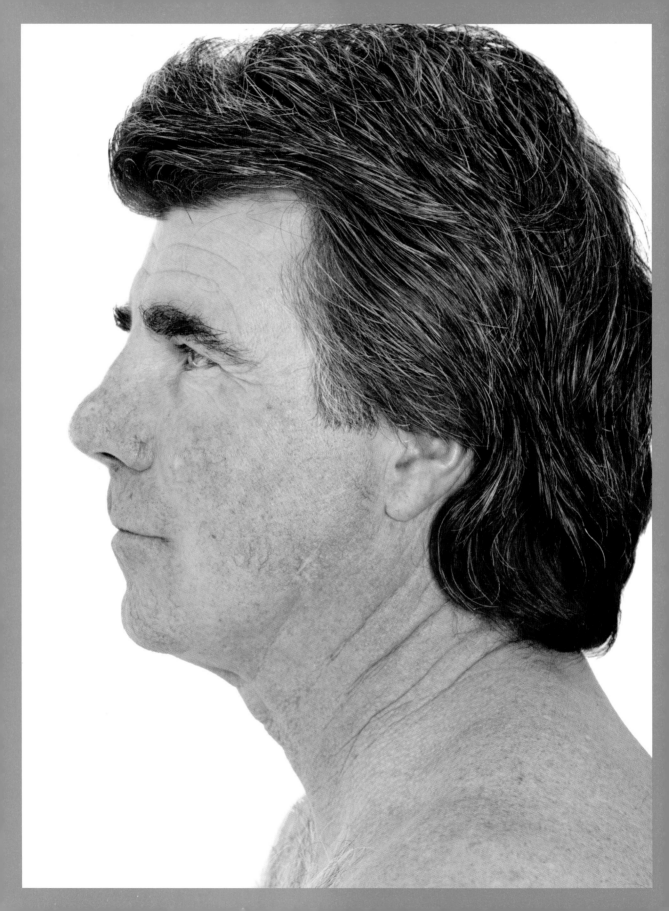

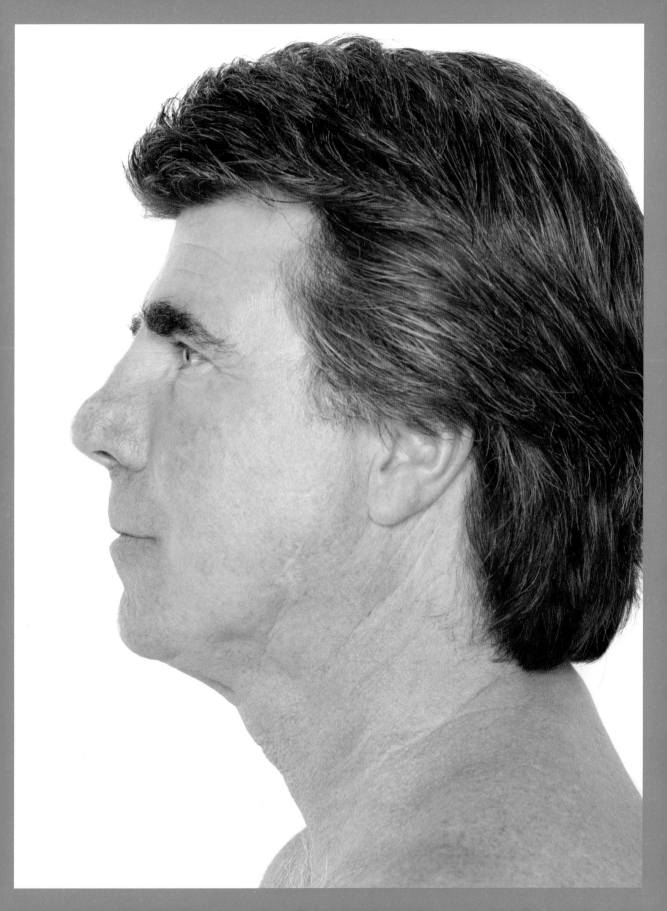

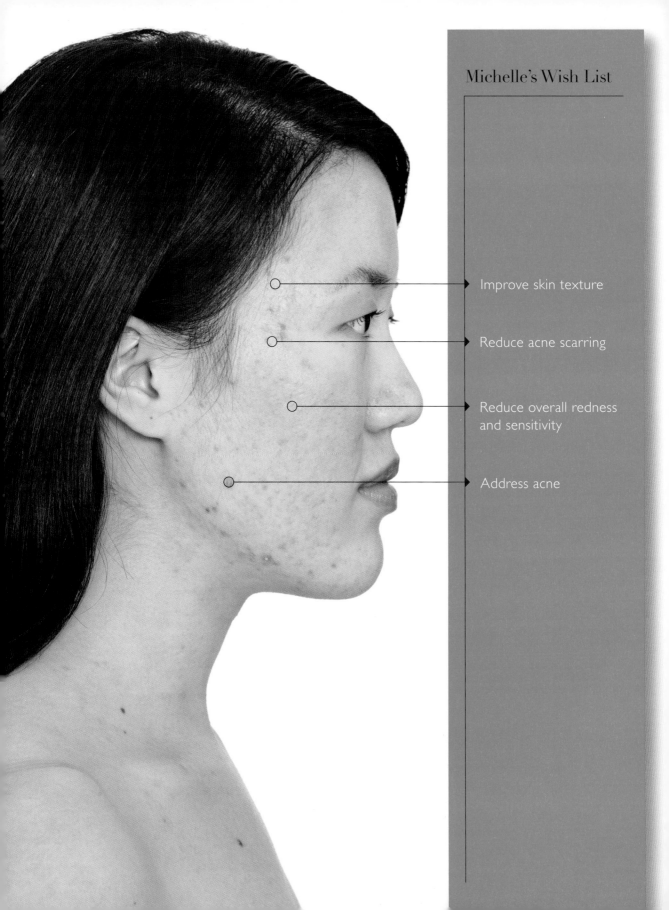

Michelle's Wish List

Improve skin texture

Reduce acne scarring

Reduce overall redness and sensitivity

Address acne

Acne, sensitivity

Michelle let me know that she's had acne since the fifth grade—perhaps it was a legacy from her dad, who had bad skin.

She'd recently gone on birth control pills, which had helped clear things up a bit, but she was still getting outbreaks around the sides of her face. This business student at USC also often studies late into the night and tends to get stressed-out during tests. Getting nervous exacerbates her skin problems, which leads to her feeling self-conscious.

In addition, Michelle explained, "My skin is very sensitive to light. Even the drive over today made it a bit red." And, she said, "I won't go outside without makeup, which takes up an extra ten minutes in the morning. I'd like an easier routine. Right now I have such a strict regimen that it's a real hassle sometimes . . . and it's expensive, too. I just want things to be simpler."

Although Michelle wanted to get rid of her acne, she had a philosophical outlook: "It's never as bad as you think it is. When I look in the mirror, I see huge pimples and redness, but when my friends talk about my skin, they'll say that they never even noticed. Sometimes it disappears in their eyes." My plan was to make it disappear in hers as well.

My Analysis

Michelle is one of those people with different ecosystems on her face. She needs to treat her acne areas separately from the rest of her skin, which is quite sensitive.

When looking at her straight on, she appears to have a perfect complexion, but the side view is another matter. Because of her sensitivity, we watched her carefully to make sure that she didn't get irritated from anything we had her using. I knew that this young lady would respond really well to the light treatments and that we'd have her superclear pretty quickly.

PRODUCTS

Step 1: Cleanse

- Detox Daily Cleanser morning and night

- Clarifying Treatment Toner on acne area

Step 2: Exfoliate

- ExfoliKate Intensive Exfoliating Treatment twice a week, all over her face

- Clearing Mask once a week, just on the acne area

Step 3: Treat

- Anti Bac Clearing Lotion twice a day, only on breakout areas

Step 4: Moisturize

- Oil Free Moisturizer morning and night

Step 5: Protect

- Protect SPF 55 Serum Sunscreen

- Omnilux™ LED anti-acne series (blue/red light); Omnilux white LED light
- Laser Genesis®
- Pearl®

- Take my Total Vitamin Clear Skin Supplement

The Results

I love to see this: Michelle was someone who once couldn't get her breakouts to stop, but with the right treatment, it was pretty easy to change that. "The texture is so much better, and the redness is barely there," she stated. "The Pearl gave me new skin! Now when I go to class or do errands, I get ready so quickly, and I'm really, really happy. I don't have to fuss with my skin anymore." She said this with a huge smile on her face.

In addition, Michelle learned how to properly take care of her skin. When she gets a minor breakout these days, she's discovered that the technique of using acne-treatment products only on the problem areas, and not on the rest of her face, really works for her sensitive skin.

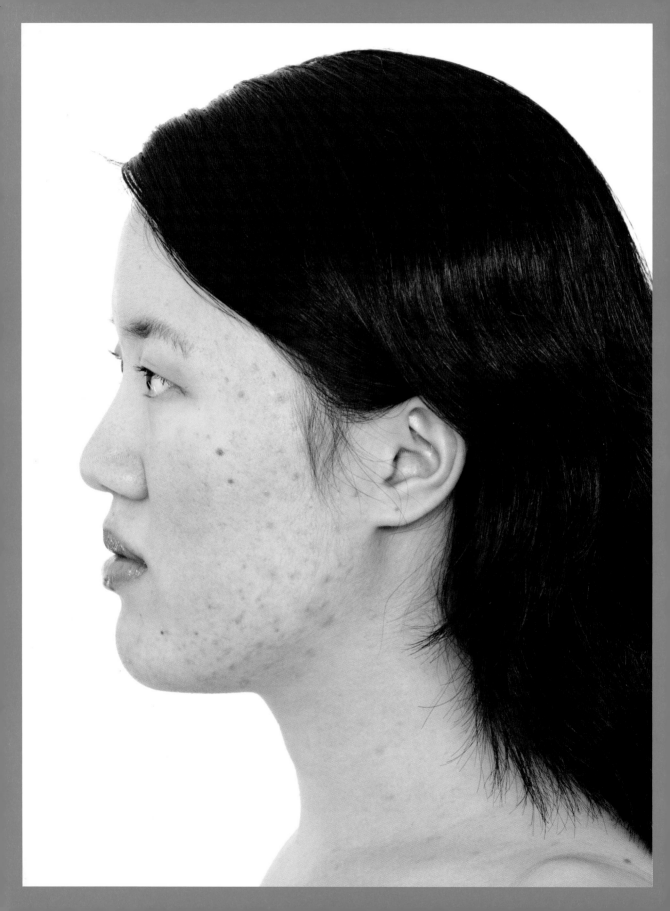

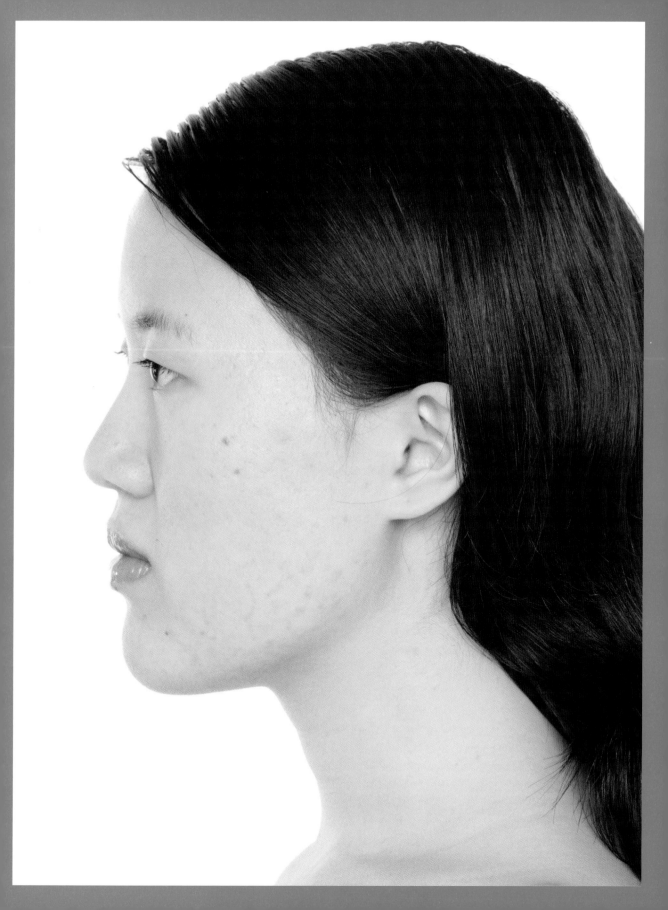

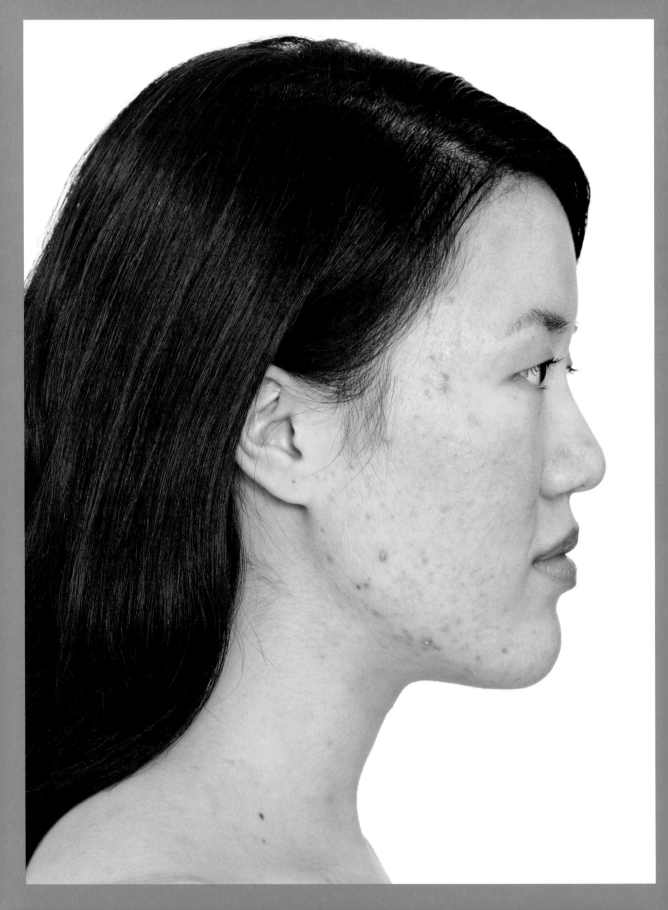

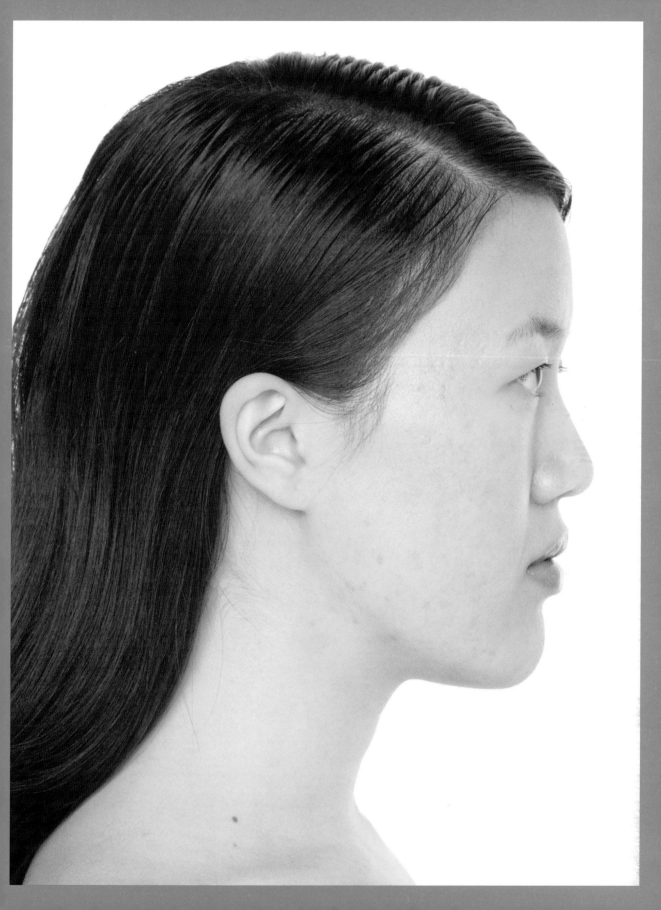

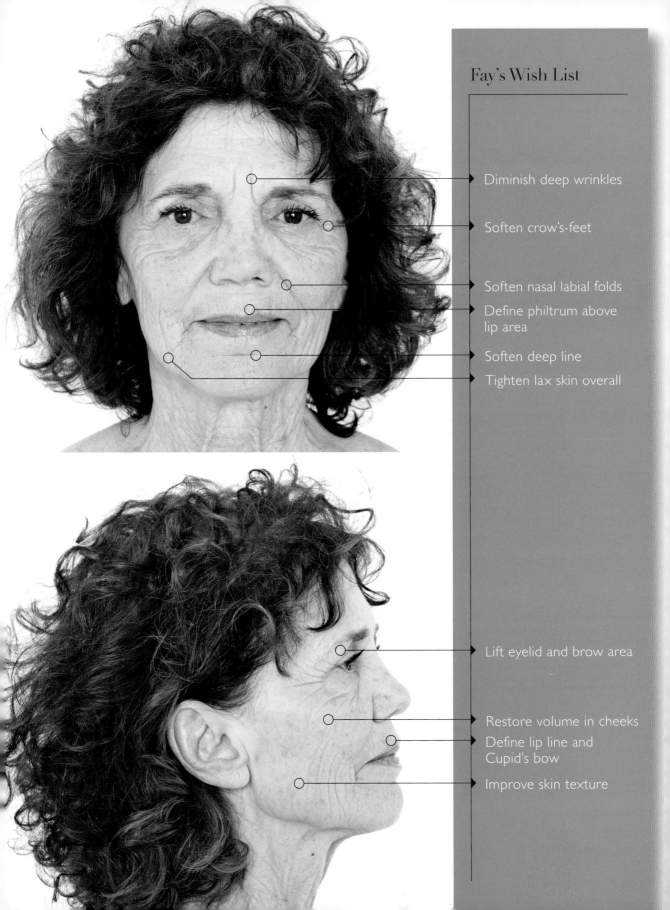

Fay's Wish List

Diminish deep wrinkles

Soften crow's-feet

Soften nasal labial folds

Define philtrum above lip area

Soften deep line

Tighten lax skin overall

Lift eyelid and brow area

Restore volume in cheeks

Define lip line and Cupid's bow

Improve skin texture

Anti-aging

Fay and her husband of 49 years own a pottery and fountainware business in Glendale, California, where she also grew up. Get this—as a girl, she'd use that old cocktail of baby oil and iodine in search of the beach-babe bronze!

As a teen, Fay was lucky and didn't have breakouts. However, she got hit with acne after her third baby was born, when she was in her 30s. She went to a dermatologist and got antibiotic shots, which was all that was available 40 years ago.

Fay has had a fair amount of stress in her life, including raising a grandchild and taking care of her 91-year-old mother. She's noticed that stress makes her skin drier and causes her to lose weight, which also shows in her face. While she had a lot of expression lines, she told me, "I don't mind my smile lines. I just don't like the ones that make me look stressed and tired." It bothered her to look in the mirror and think, *I wish I didn't have all this.* She said, "I'd like to look on the outside like I feel on the inside." That is something most of us can identify with as we get older.

My Analysis

I promised Fay this: "I can give you that radiance back, so when you look in the mirror, you're not going to feel disappointed. You're going to feel good about yourself."

Fay has the kind of skin that shows results pretty quickly. I didn't see a huge amount of sun damage; it was primarily skin laxity, so that is what we decided to concentrate on. She mostly needed laser therapies with a little bit of Botox for expression lines and fillers. She had a beautiful mouth, so I wanted to bring it back to life by using fillers in the philtrum and the lip line. She's already gorgeous—my goal wasn't to make her look 30 years younger, but to bring that vibrancy and glow back into her face, soften the deep lines, and just tighten her up.

PRODUCTS

Step 1: Cleanse

- Gentle Daily Wash morning and night

Step 2: Exfoliate

- ExfoliKate Intensive Exfoliating Treatment twice a week

Step 3: Treat

- Total Vitamin Antioxidant Complex and Quench Hydrating Face Serum morning and night

Step 4: Moisturize

- Deep Tissue Repair Cream and Line Release Under Eye Repair Cream morning and night

Step 5: Protect

- Protect SPF 55 Serum Sunscreen

- Titan®
- Pearl®
- Laser Genesis®
- Botox®
- Juvéderm®

- Restylane®
- Radiesse®
- Omnilux™ white and red LED lights
- Muscle Lift
- CoolGlide Vascular Therapy

DIET AND LIFESTYLE RECOMMENDATION

- Fay already practices a very healthy lifestyle and takes an impressive array of supplements, including hyaluronic acid. She works out regularly—always has, she says—and practices stretching and meditation. Therefore, I didn't need to offer her any suggestions here.

The Results

"I feel beautiful!" Fay declared after finishing her treatment program. She was now starting her mornings feeling better about herself and more excited about the day ahead: "I wake up and look in the mirror, and I'm so happy." She said that she no longer looked stressed or tired and that she got the results she wanted: to look the way she felt inside. She also reported that she'd ditched her normal makeup routine—she didn't need as much because her skin was so evenly toned and the texture had significantly improved.

Fay told me that her husband, a man of few words, thought she looked amazing and that neighbors and friends all commented on how wonderful she looks. "One person even asked me if I'd had a face-lift!" she said. She commented that she hadn't had a pampered life, but from now on, she would definitely keep up a program of skin care and treatments.

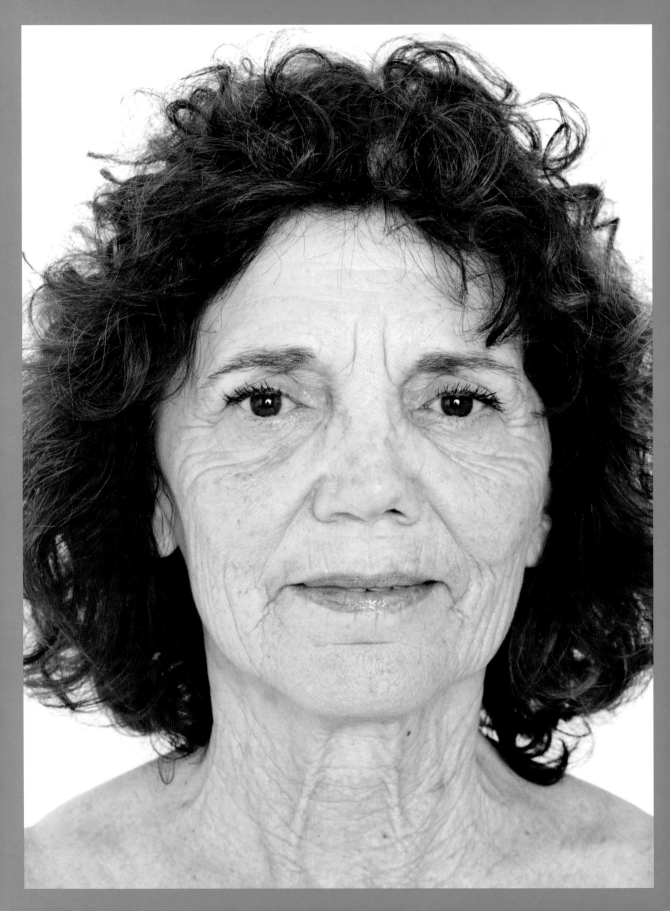

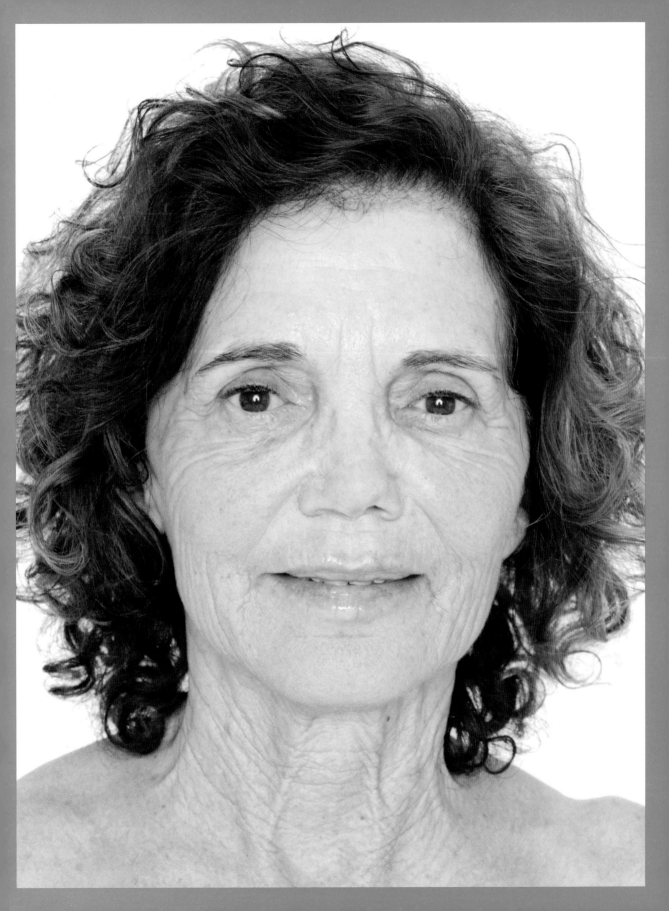

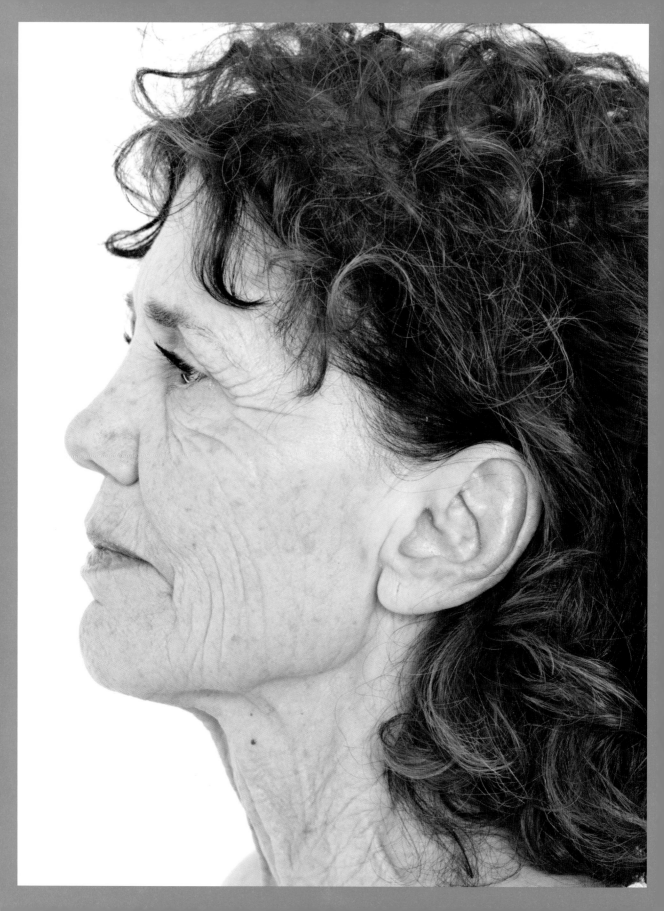

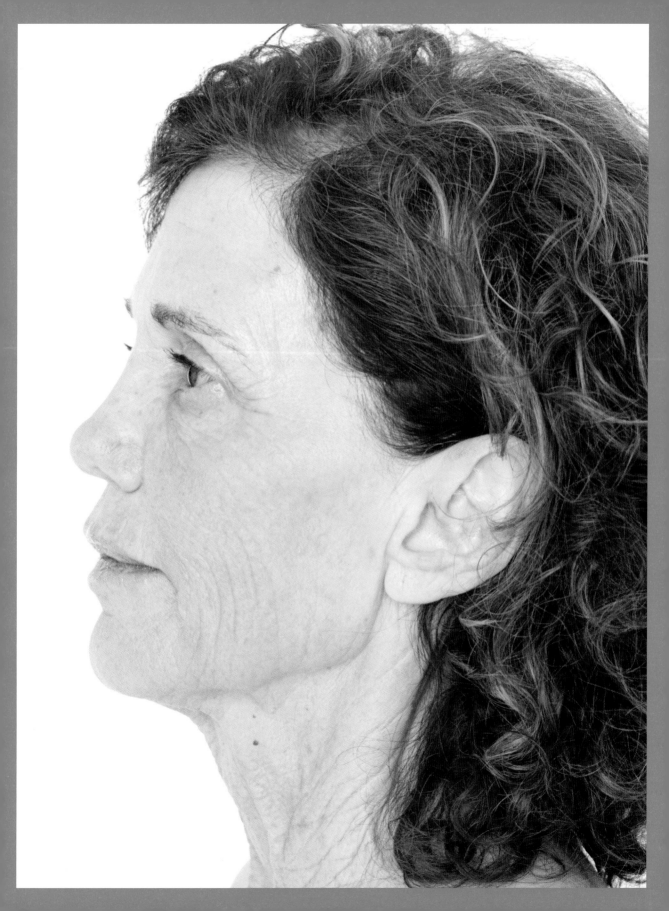

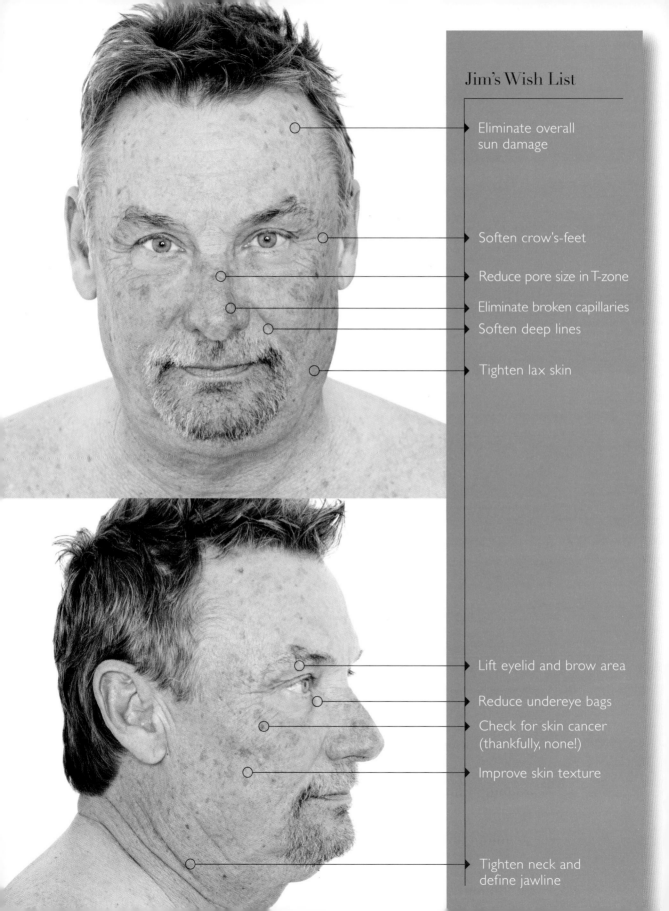

Jim's Wish List

Eliminate overall
sun damage

Soften crow's-feet

Reduce pore size in T-zone

Eliminate broken capillaries

Soften deep lines

Tighten lax skin

Lift eyelid and brow area

Reduce undereye bags

Check for skin cancer
(thankfully, none!)

Improve skin texture

Tighten neck and
define jawline

Anti-aging, sun damage

My husband and I have known Jim for a long time—he used to be our neighbor and is now our friend—and I was so excited to finally get my hands on his skin!

Jim is a native Texan and a real outdoorsman who loves to fish. (Fishing actually increases sun exposure, as the water reflects UV rays.) He's also a movie producer who's generally on location, shooting outdoors. He told me that he tried to wear sunscreen, but I wasn't really convinced.

Jim is a guy's guy who wasn't worried about his skin, but he did say that it looked a lot better when he was younger. I wanted to give him back a few years.

My Analysis

My friend obviously had a lot of sun damage. He also had some discoloration on his cheek that my team and I felt needed to be seen by a dermatologist, so we referred him to someone before we started treatments. It turned out to be nothing, so we were able to proceed with no problems.

Jim didn't really do anything for his skin, so this whole process was totally new to him. I let him know that if we were going to get rid of his sun damage and restore a healthier complexion, he'd have to do his part. He promised he would—and since he's such a great person, I knew that he'd be up for the challenge.

PRODUCTS

Step 1: Cleanse

- Gentle Daily Wash morning and night

Step 2: Exfoliate

- ExfoliKate Intensive Exfoliating Treatment twice a week

Step 3: Treat

- Quench Hydrating Face Serum morning and night

Step 4: Moisturize

- Deep Tissue Repair Cream morning and night

Step 5: Protect

- Protect SPF 55 Serum Sunscreen

CLINIC TREATMENTS

- Laser Genesis®
- Titan®
- Pearl®
- IPL
- Hyfrecator for skin tags
- CoolGlide Vascular Therapy
- TCA peel
- Omnilux™ white and red LED lights

The Results

Jim's results just blew us all away—including him! When I saw him after his last treatment, I actually laughed at what I'd put him through. Coming in for facials and lights and lasers . . . but man, he looked good! We literally cleaned his face up and took years off of his skin so that he looked at least a decade younger. And believe it or not, we also found a skin cancer while he was undergoing services with us. We sent him to a doctor to have it treated.

"I'm thrilled to death with what you've done," Jim reported. "Honestly, I never expected this difference." Everyone's noticing how great he looks, and it's been fun to see him get this attention.

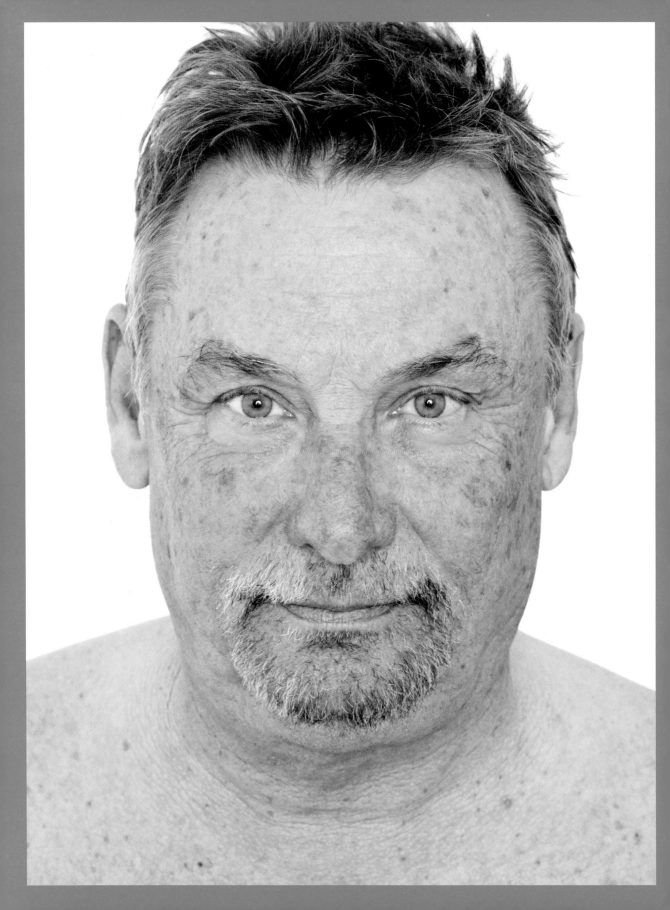

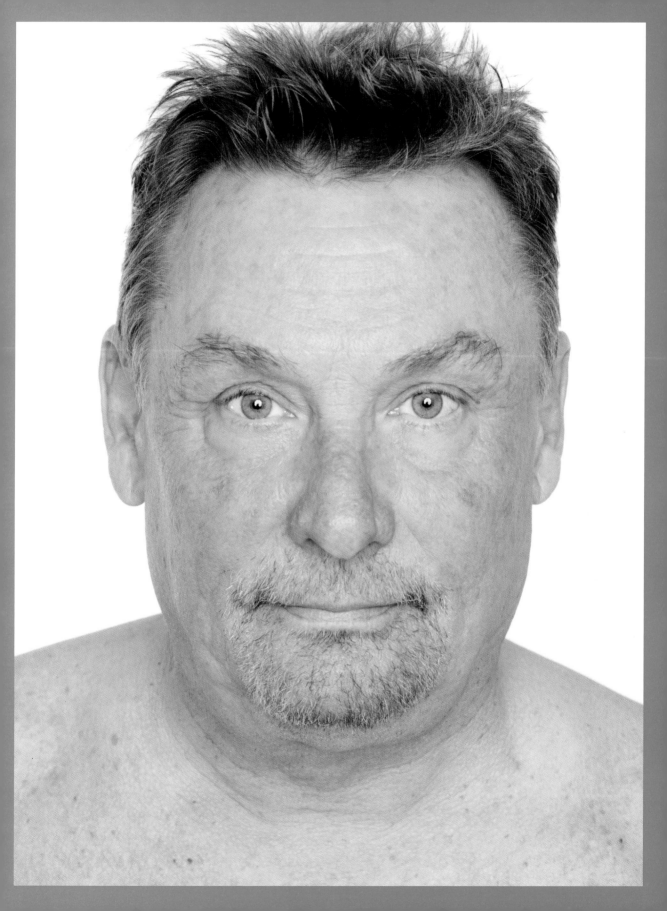

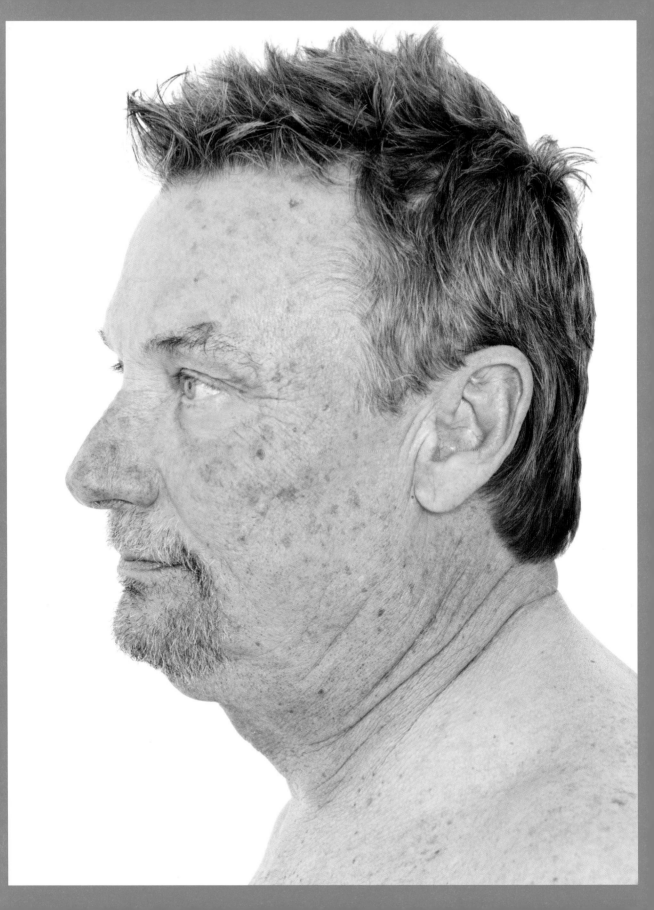

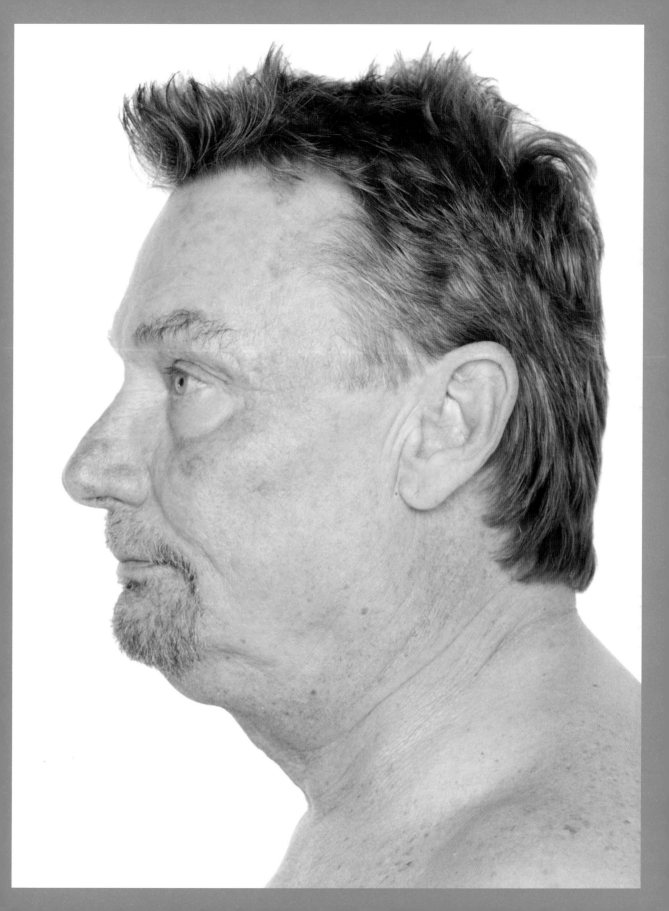

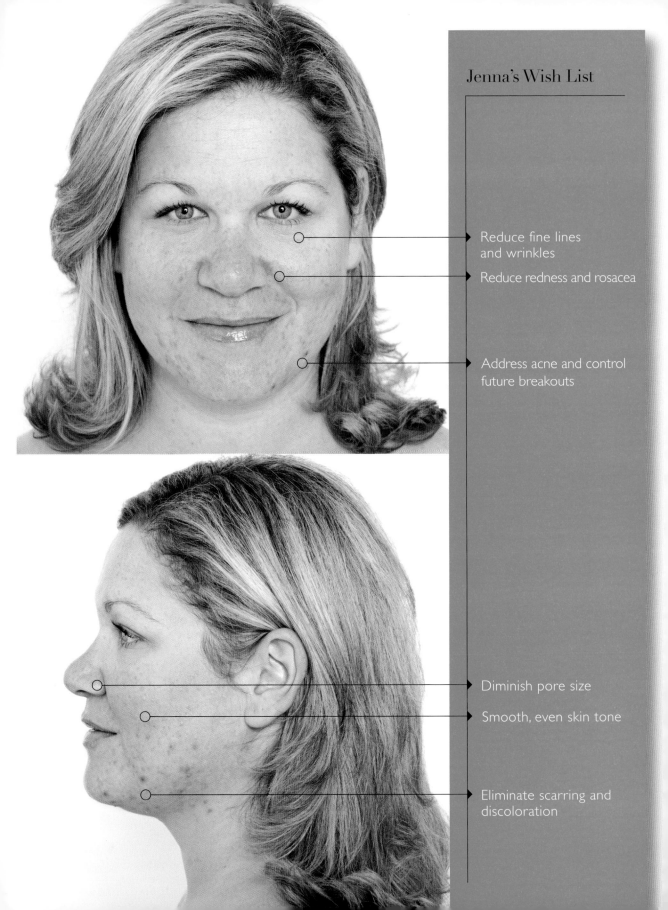

Jenna's Wish List

Reduce fine lines
and wrinkles

Reduce redness and rosacea

Address acne and control
future breakouts

Diminish pore size

Smooth, even skin tone

Eliminate scarring and
discoloration

Acne, scarring, discoloration, T-zone oiliness

Jenna lives in West Los Angeles and is beginning her Ph.D. program at Texas A&M University. Congratulations, Jenna! She's excited, as you might expect, and wants to start this new chapter of her life with a clear complexion.

When Jenna came in, she believed that her main skin problem was her adult-onset acne, mostly along her jaw and neck area. She said that she first started getting it at age 25, when she was working like mad in a very stressful job, with 80-hour weeks and travel all over, which led to lack of sleep and a poor diet. (I can totally relate.)

"I've been to dermatologists and tried pretty much everything under the sun for my acne: over-the-counter benzoyl peroxide products, Retin-A, antibiotic pills," Jenna let me know, "but nothing's really helped. In fact, I think that some things even made it worse."

This young woman felt extremely self-conscious about her skin. She wore a lot of makeup to try to cover it up, but she knew that the acne was still there, and she thought that everyone could see it. She said that it negatively impacted her social life: "I used to be pretty vivacious and outgoing. I'd like to be that person again, and I feel that I could be, if I were just more comfortable with my skin and the way I look." Although she's single, she admitted, "I don't put myself out there like I should because I don't feel pretty. Even in intimate situations, I feel very self-conscious and uncomfortable with people touching my face because I feel like I'm not attractive."

My Analysis

Jenna had moderate acne, as well as scarring from old outbreaks. I also saw some texture problems, including enlarged pores, a little bit of rosacea, some patches of discoloration, and sun damage. Her nose was red and shiny, which I believe was the result of many severe sunburns. She had an oily T-zone, too.

Skin that has so much going on needs a multipronged approach. My plan was to regulate Jenna's complexion with several products, which would give her results that she could see and feel. I also felt that it was necessary to use treatments that would go a lot deeper to handle the scarring and skin texture.

PRODUCTS

Step 1: Cleanse

- Detox Daily Cleanser in the morning

- Purify Exfoliating Cleanser and Clarifying Treatment Toner at night

Step 2: Exfoliate

- ExfoliKate Intensive Exfoliating Treatment twice a week

- Clearing Mask once a week; should also be left overnight on big cystic-acne outbreaks

Step 3: Treat

- Anti Bac Clearing Lotion twice a day, only on breakout areas

Step 4: Moisturize

- Oil Free Moisturizer and Line Release Under Eye Repair Cream morning and night

CLINIC TREATMENTS

- Omnilux™ LED anti-acne and anti-aging series (one series of blue/red; one series of white/red)
- Titan®, just in the acne-scarred area
- Pearl®

- Laser Genesis®
- IPL
- Restylane®, just in acne scars
- Botox®

DIET AND LIFESTYLE RECOMMENDATIONS

- Stay off of dairy and soy products; replace with rice or almond milk

- Reduce sugar, white bread, and pasta intake

- Take my Total Vitamin Clear Skin Supplement

The Results

After ten weeks, my team was able to get rid of most of Jenna's acne, and she's not having breakouts like she did before. Also, the texture of her skin is smoother and softer and more evenly toned. She's wearing a lot less makeup and has switched to a mineral foundation that gives her sheerer coverage. As she told me, "My skin is looking a hundred times better! I feel more comfortable and confident going out now, and I'm not embarrassed to talk to people or get too close to them. And I'm getting a lot of compliments from my friends!"

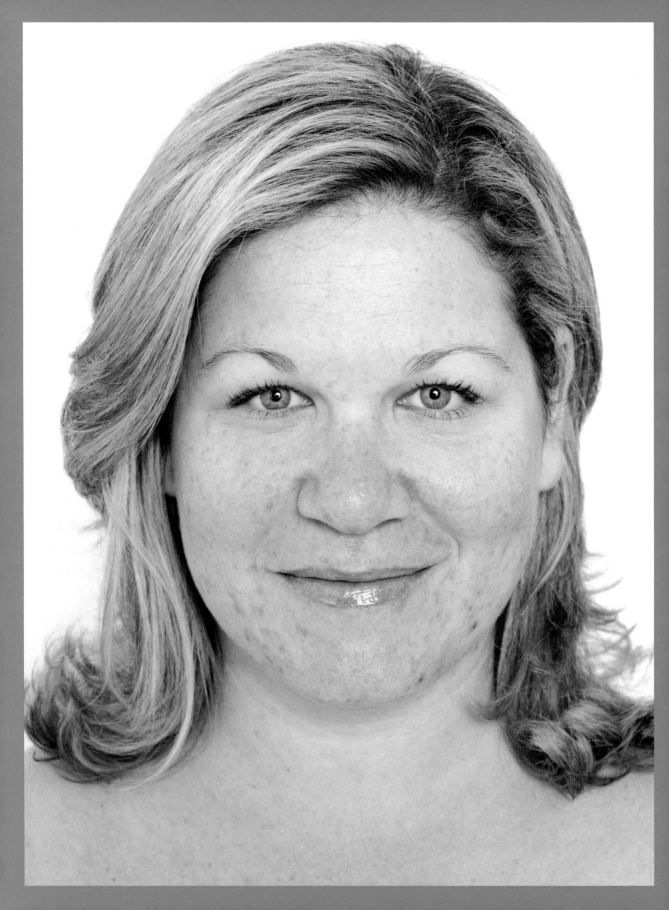

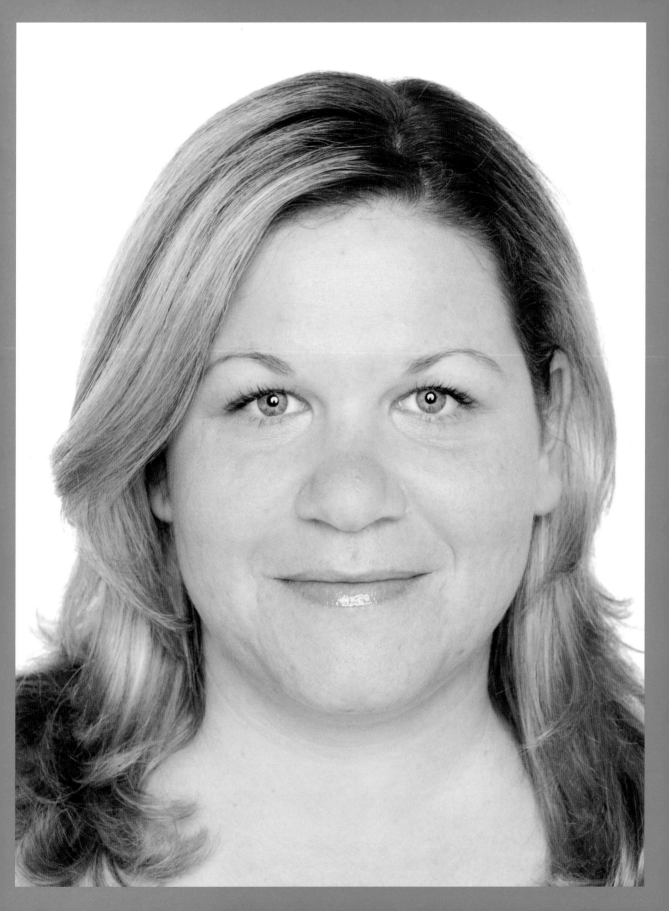

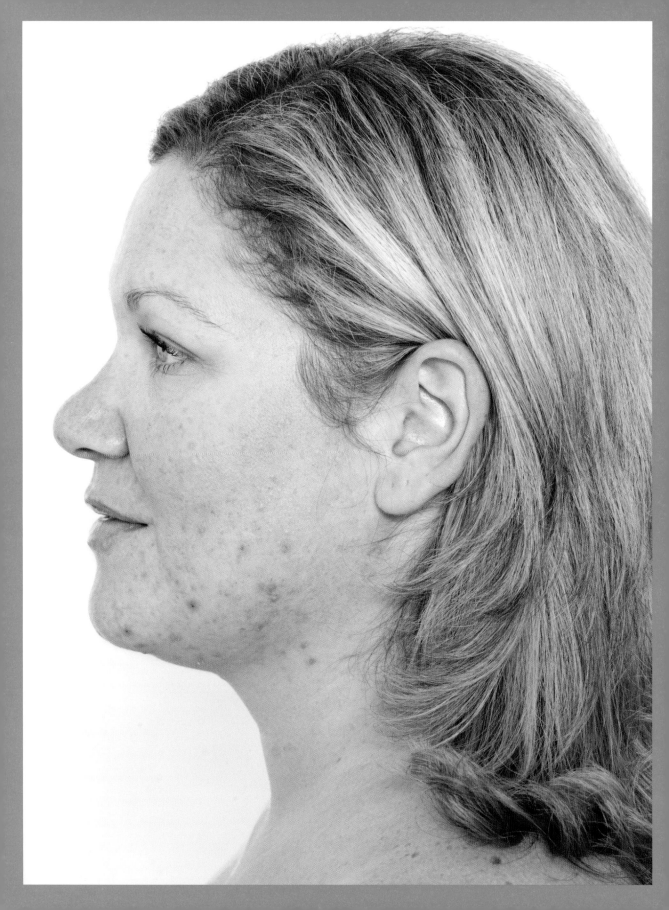

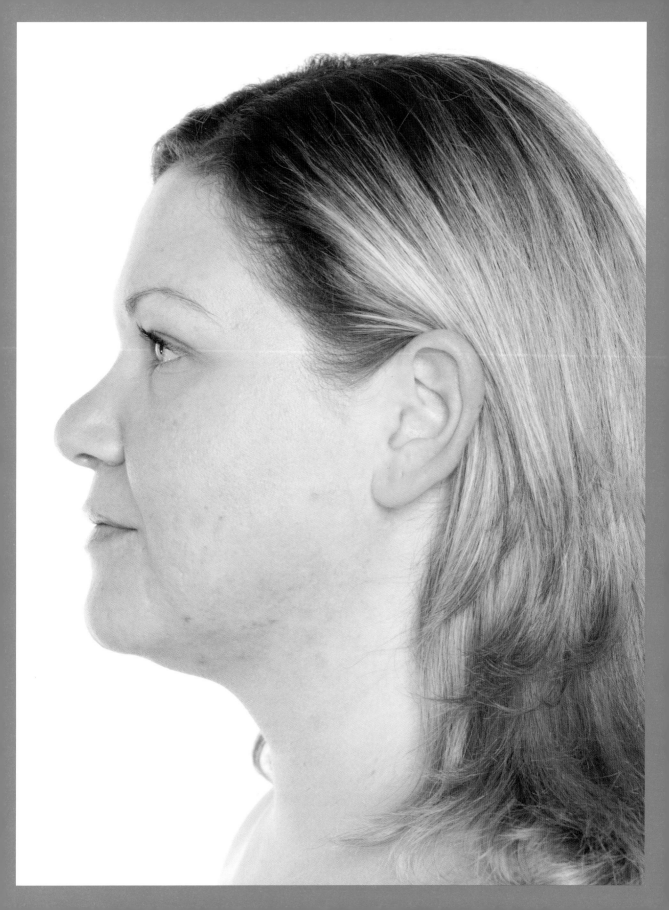

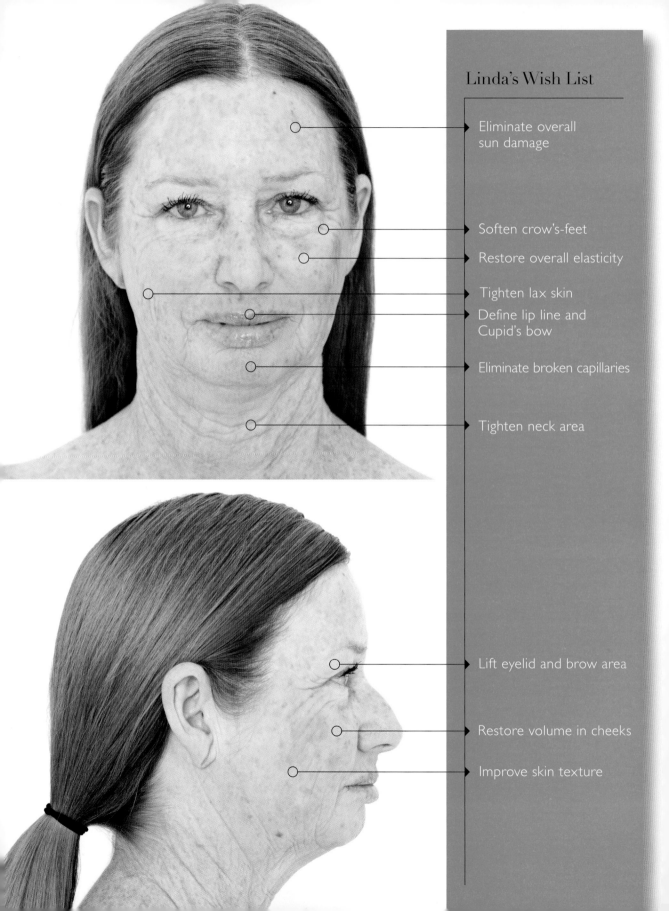

Linda's Wish List

Eliminate overall sun damage

Soften crow's-feet

Restore overall elasticity

Tighten lax skin

Define lip line and Cupid's bow

Eliminate broken capillaries

Tighten neck area

Lift eyelid and brow area

Restore volume in cheeks

Improve skin texture

Anti-aging, pigmentation

Linda, who inherited fair, Celtic-type skin from her Scottish mother, showed up for her "before" pictures in jodhpurs. She's a big-time horsewoman who rides as often as she can, and she's always spent a lot of time outside. Although she insisted that she "never wanted to do the baby-oil thing to try to get tan," she also admitted that she hadn't always used sun protection.

Linda told me that about 20 years ago, she became more knowledgeable about skin care and tried everything on her skin, including some of the most expensive brands on the market. Unfortunately, she hadn't seen the results she'd been looking for, and for the last ten years or so, she'd been feeling very self-conscious and insecure. In fact, she'd become so unhappy with her appearance that she tried to cover her face as much as possible with her long hair.

I met Linda on the set of QVC, where she often travels with her colleague Chaz Dean, who sells his incredible line of hair-care products there. She told me that she'd purchased my Quench Hydrating Serum: "I thought it was the holy grail, and I'm hooked on it." She'd already seen results from using it for a couple of months, so I was looking forward to introducing her to my other products and treatments. My plan was for Linda's skin to be as healthy and stunning as her hair was!

My Analysis

Linda had significant sun damage, and there was more of it on her left side. (This is common in the U.S., since we tend to get a lot more sun through the car window while we're driving.) She was also exhibiting signs of aging and laxity, along with pretty deep expression lines. But with a combo of laser treatments and injectables, we'd have her looking younger and feeling more confident in just a few short weeks.

PRODUCTS

Step 1: Cleanse

- Gentle Daily Wash in the morning

Step 2: Exfoliate

- ExfoliKate Intensive Exfoliating Treatment twice a week

Step 3: Treat

- Total Vitamin Antioxidant Complex and Quench Hydrating Face Serum morning and night

Step 4: Moisturize

- Deep Tissue Repair Cream and Line Release Under Eye Repair Cream morning and night

Step 5: Protect

- Protect SPF 55 Serum Sunscreen

- Titan®
- Pearl®
- Laser Genesis®
- CoolGlide Vascular Therapy
- Omnilux™ white and red LED lights
- IPL

- Botox®
- Restylane®
- Radiesse®
- Juvéderm®
- TCA peel

The Results

Linda's results have been truly transformative. When I saw her after the treatments were finished, she made me cry. She told me that she felt so confident about herself that when Chaz asked her to go on TV with him as a hair model, she actually said, "Yes!" She claimed that there was no way she would have ever done this before, not even when she was younger. When I asked her what she loved most about the makeover process, she said, "I have my lips back! The results are dramatic, but still subtle."

A few days later, at a big beauty event, women guessed Linda's age to be 10 to 12 years younger, and people were asking her what products she's using, not what she'd had done. Now her skin truly is as lovely and as healthy as her hair.

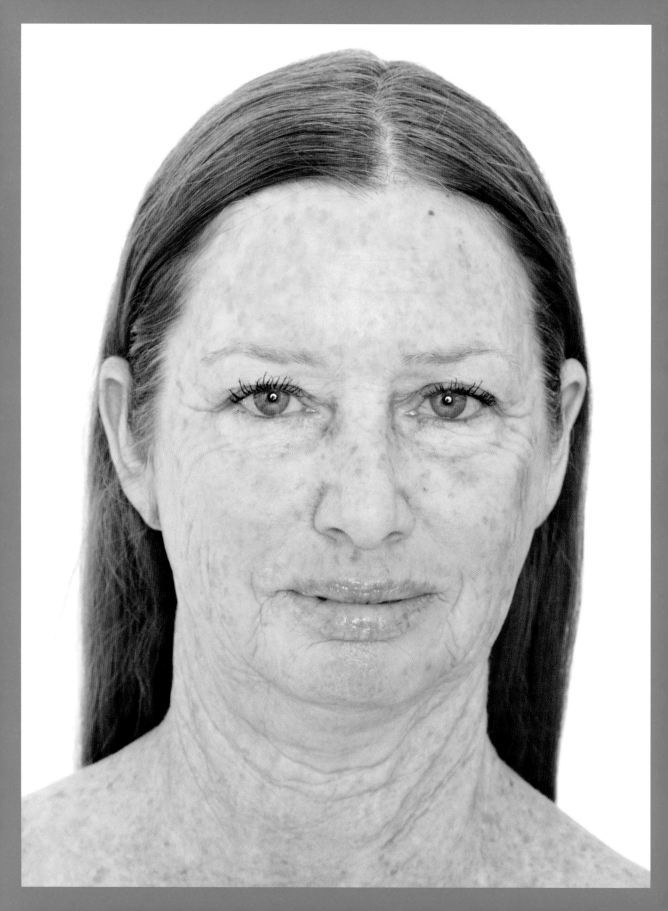

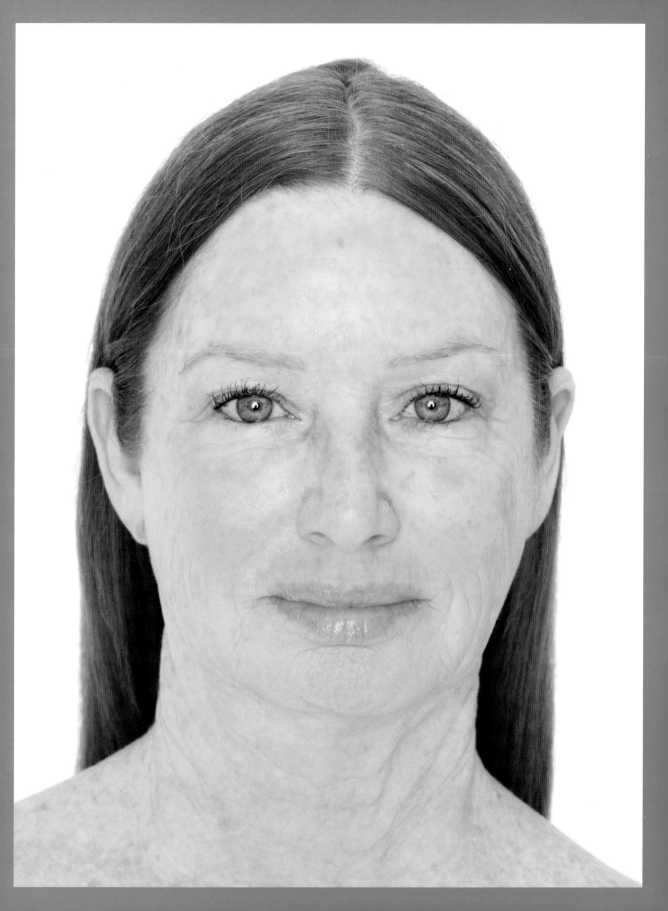

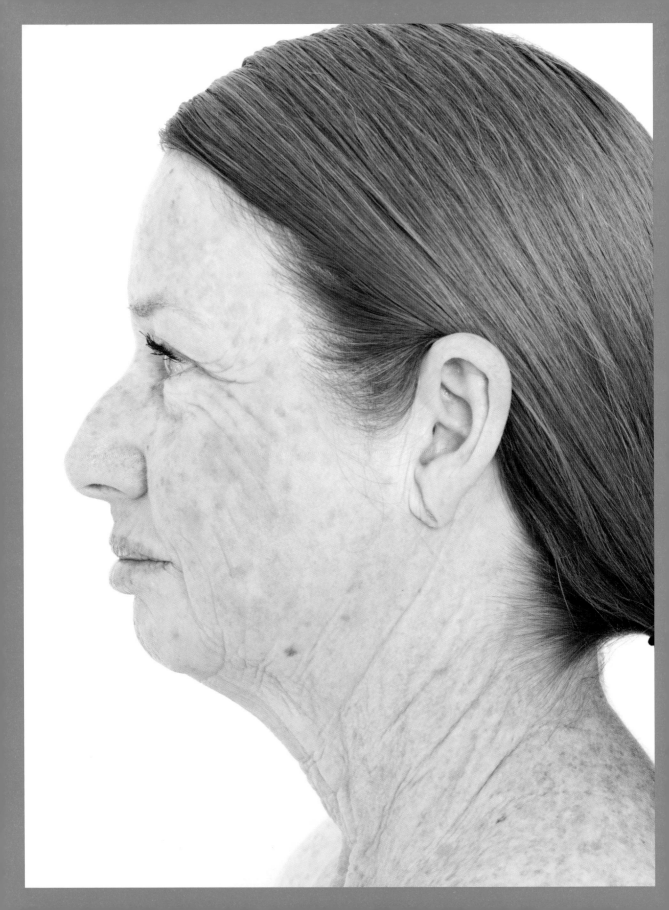

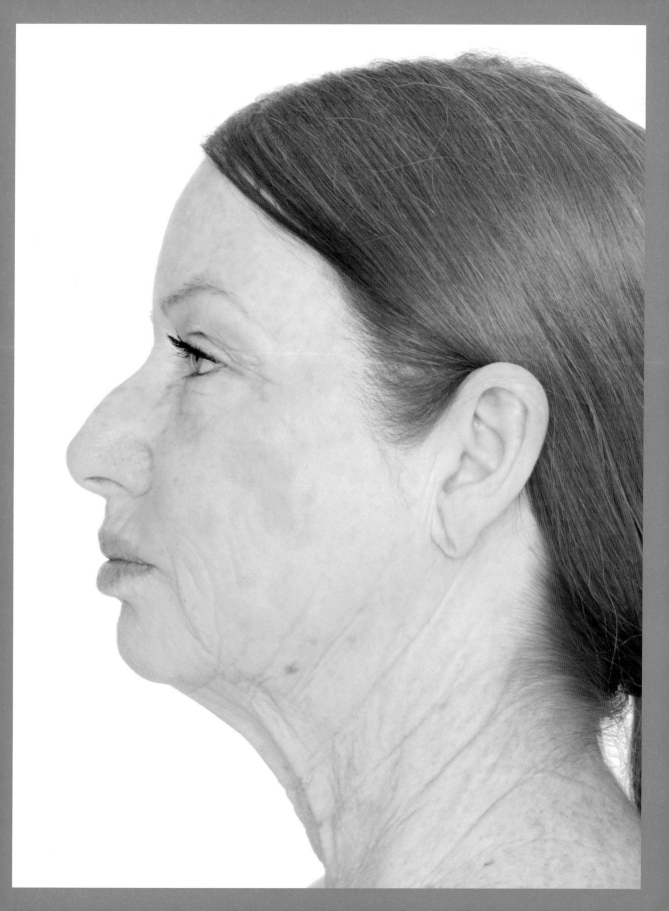

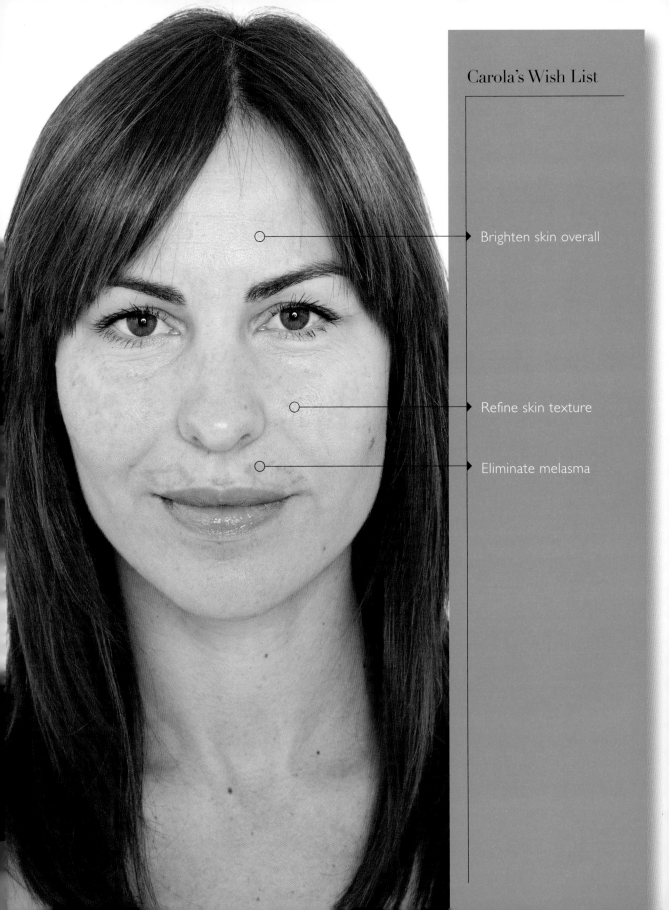

Carola's Wish List

Brighten skin overall

Refine skin texture

Eliminate melasma

Melasma

Carola, an existing client of mine, is a former model who's now a professional makeup artist. Over the years, she's sent a lot of her celebrities to my clinic. My team and I have worked on their skin and on hers as well.

Overall, Carola has gorgeous skin. She treats it well, coming to see us regularly for facials and caring for it herself. "I believe that your skin talks to you," she likes to say, echoing my own philosophy. But when you look closely at her skin, she has dark pigment and discoloration above her lip and on her cheeks. She said that she was tired of covering her "melasma mustache" with makeup and just wanted to get rid of it. She told me that she'd gotten it to fade in the past with topical creams, but it always came back. I knew we had to get to the bottom of the melasma, or else it would always be there—so that was my main goal.

My Analysis

Carola has beautiful skin, but this blotchy band of pigment above her lip was distracting. I'm still not sure what was causing her melasma, which she said appeared when she was about 30. In most cases, pigmentation comes from either injury or hormonal changes, and above-the-lip melasma tends to be a solid band. Since Carola's was a wavy line, one possibility is that she might have been injured by waxing there; because of the age she was when it appeared, it could also be due to hormones. As for the spots near her cheeks, these were most likely the result of lots of sun, as she had grown up in Puerto Rico.

I was confident that with minor treatment and topical products, we could fix any discoloration. Carola's was a pretty simple case, and very common.

PRODUCTS

Step 1: Cleanse

- Gentle Daily Wash morning and night

Step 2: Exfoliate

- ExfoliKate Intensive Exfoliating Treatment twice a week

Step 3: Treat

- Refrigerator Cream daily for two weeks: I instructed Carola to use a Q-tip to push the cream just into the discolored area. She needed to avoid the skin that was not dis-colored in order to keep it from lightening up. I told her to take a break from the cream after we did the Pearl, until her skin recovered from the peel.

Step 4: Moisturize

■ Total Vitamin Antioxidant Complex and Quench Hydrating Face Serum morning and night

Step 5: Protect

■ Protect SPF 30 Sunscreen

■ Omnilux™ white and red LED lights

■ Pearl®
■ Laser Genesis®

■ Take my Total Vitamin Anti-Aging Supplement

The Results

Carola's melasma was much improved, but she still needs some ongoing treatment. I'm going to have her continue using the cream and maybe do one more Pearl to totally knock out the rest of the pigment. Overall, though, Carola's complexion brightened and tightened. She loved the results and was thrilled to see the changes happening before her eyes. "The texture is better and my skin is much smoother," she told me. "I definitely see a difference in my pore size. And I'm so happy that the pigment above my lip is almost gone!"

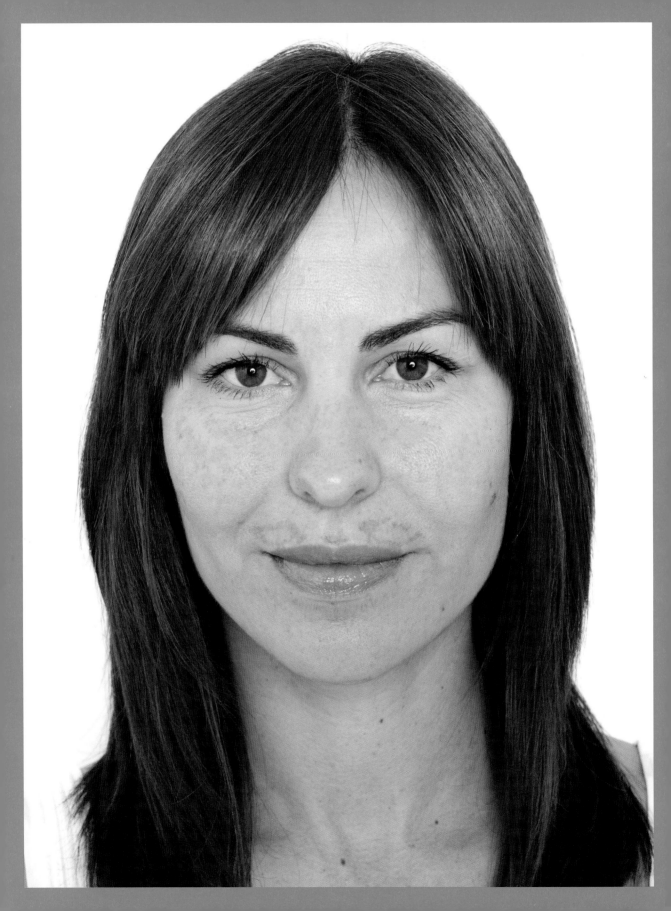

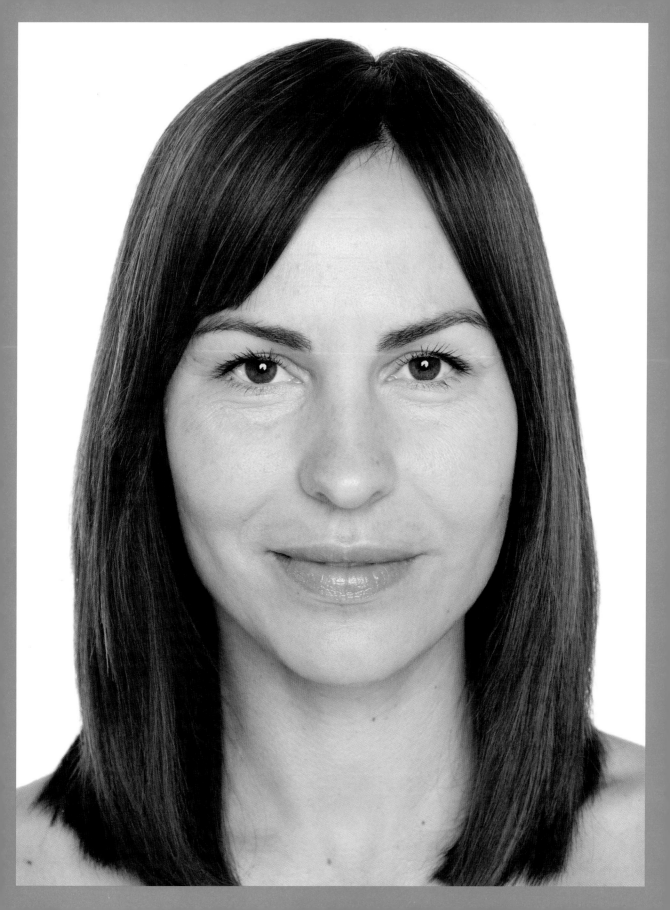

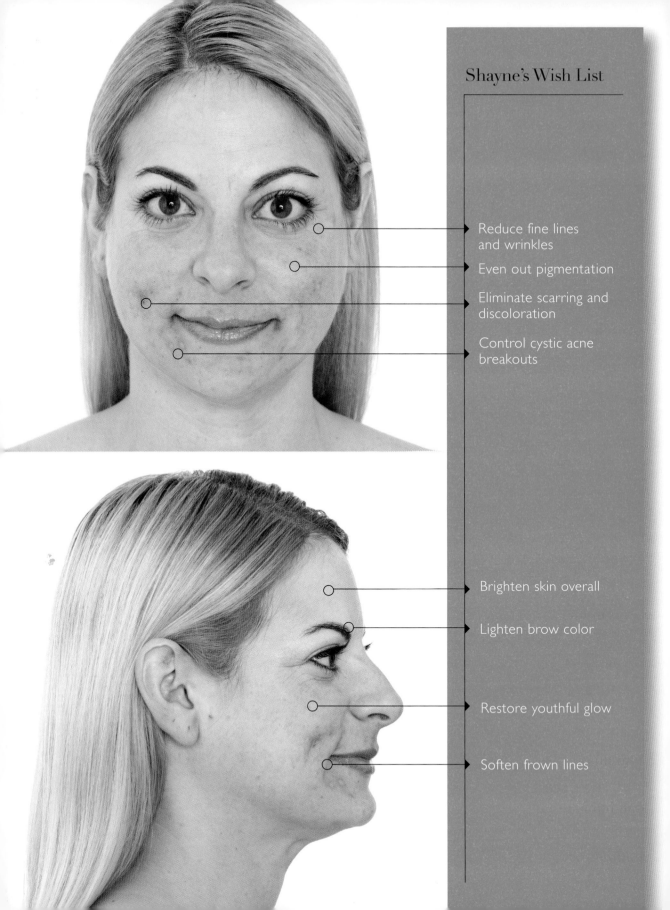

Shayne's Wish List

Reduce fine lines and wrinkles

Even out pigmentation

Eliminate scarring and discoloration

Control cystic acne breakouts

Brighten skin overall

Lighten brow color

Restore youthful glow

Soften frown lines

Cystic acne, post-acne scarring, anti-aging, dryness

Shayne has a master's degree in education, and she's also a second-generation psychic. Both she and her sister have the "gift," which was passed along to them by their mom. "Ever since I was little, I've been able to look at people and know things," Shayne explained when we met. So recently she's stepped out to use this talent in different ways: she does professional events as well as personal readings and speaking engagements.

"And I do a lot of coaching for teenagers," she said. "Helping people find their direction is what it's all about." It's pretty intimate work, and to do that, she wants to put her best face forward.

Growing up in Southern California, Shayne spent a lot of time in the sun, so she had spots of dark pigmentation and aging sun damage. But what was really bothering her was her post-acne scarring. She told me that she'd gone on birth control pills to regulate her menstrual cycle at the age of 16. When she went off them some years later, she had a massive outbreak of acne on her cheeks. "I'm the nervous type, so I'd pick at the blemishes, causing scars," she said. She eventually went back on the pills, and the acne cleared up a little, but she still had scarring and the occasional cyst.

While Shayne believes that beauty comes from the inside, she also knows that everyone feels better when they think that they look better on the outside. "My skin really affects my self-esteem, and there are times when I feel very self-conscious, very insecure." So when her childhood best friend (who's a nurse at my clinic) told her about the makeover program, she was eager to volunteer.

My Analysis

Shayne was typical of a lot of my clients in that she's at that age where she thought she'd be finished with acne, but it's actually worse than ever. The kind of deep, cystic acne that leaves marks can be so frustrating. Because Shayne was also just beginning to show signs of aging, she fit into the acne/mature combination. You can't just dry the pimples out, because that strategy won't work—it will actually accelerate the signs of aging.

So the plan was to stop the acne and get rid of some of the scarring. On top of that, I wanted to diminish the lines around Shayne's eyes and forehead. Overall, I wanted to make her skin fresh and beautiful; for her, it was mainly a case of "cleaning up" the skin. But I did make her promise me that she would *not* "pick" if and when her acne flared up!

PRODUCTS

Step 1: Cleanse

- Gentle Daily Wash morning and night

Step 2: Exfoliate

- ExfoliKate Intensive Exfoliating Treatment twice a week

Step 3: Treat

- Anti Bac Clearing Lotion once a day, just when she began to feel that little knot of a cyst beginning

- Clearing Mask in the same way, leaving it on the blemish overnight

Step 4: Moisturize

- Deep Tissue Repair Cream, from her cheeks up, morning and night

- Oil Free Moisturizer, on her lower face, morning and night

- Line Release Under Eye Repair Cream morning and night

Step 5: Protect

- Protect SPF 30 Sunscreen

CLINIC TREATMENTS

- Omnilux™ LED anti-acne and anti-aging series (one series of blue/red; one series of white/red)
- Pearl®
- Titan® (on necessary areas)

- CoolGlide Vascular Therapy on fine red veins on her face
- IPL (two treatments)
- Laser Genesis®

DIET AND LIFESTYLE RECOMMENDATIONS

- Stay off dairy and soy products; replace with rice or almond milk

- Eat fish like salmon for the omega-3 fatty acids

- Have a small piece of dark chocolate, but only when she *really* needed a fix!

- Take my Total Vitamin Clear Skin Supplement

The Results

The difference in Shayne is incredible—her skin absolutely looks fresher and simply glows now. "The results are amazing," she said. "My skin is so much smoother, and a lot of the redness and pigmentation is gone." She was especially excited to see her fine lines just disappear, especially around the eyes. Other people are noticing, too, asking her what she's using on her skin. She still has the occasional cyst, but that's just hormonal. So we continue to do our best, preventing scarring and managing breakouts, or at least reducing their life span with the products listed.

"I didn't realize how much my skin affected my self-esteem negatively, and how much it's been a hindrance to me," Shayne told me. "I feel really good about myself now." That feeling gave her strength, confidence, and energy. In fact, in the time between her "before" and "after" pictures, Shayne landed a publishing deal to write a book about her life and growing up in a family of psychics. She's so excited about beginning this project with an entirely new outlook and personal strength.

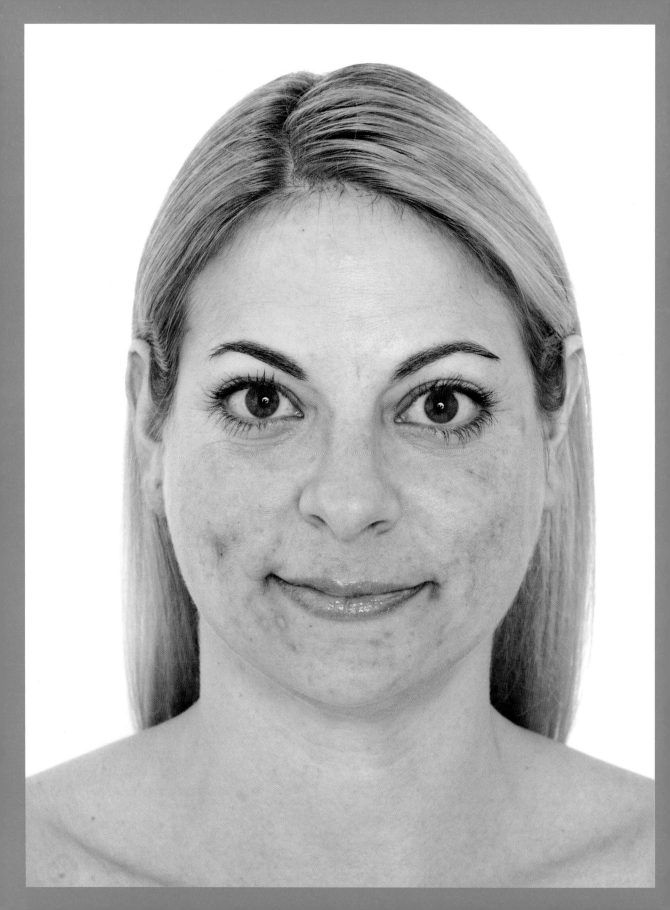

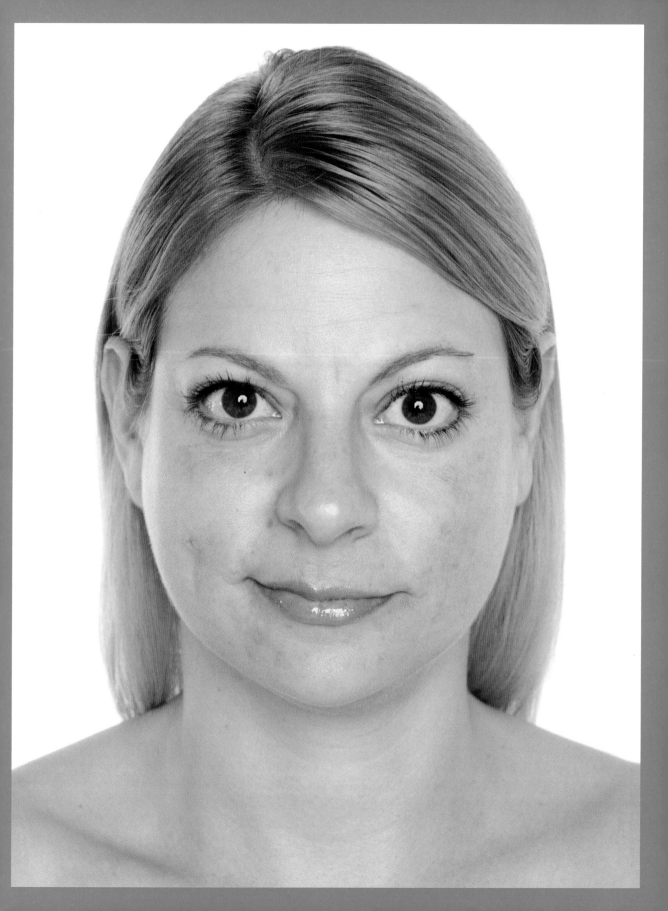

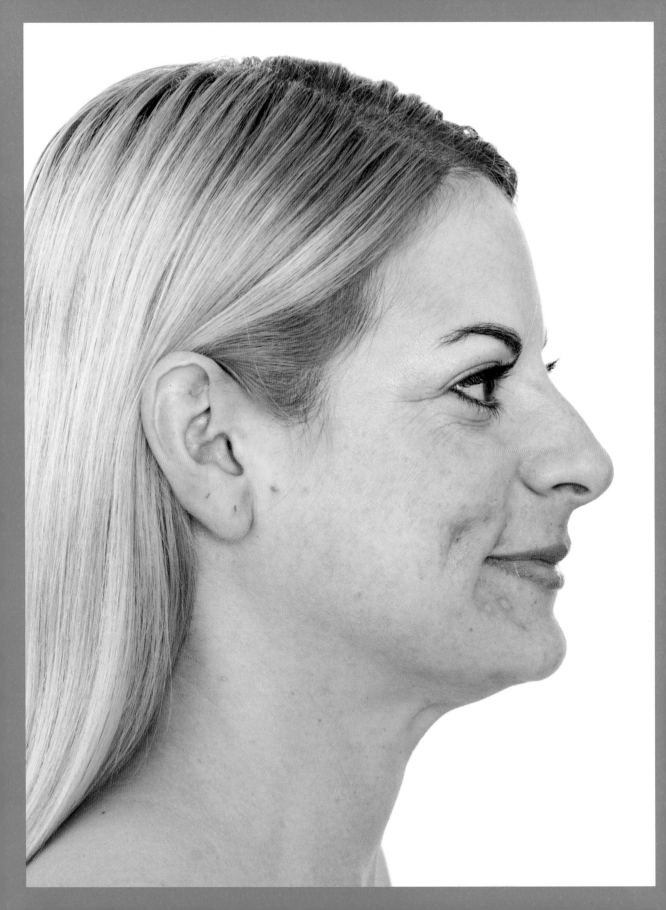

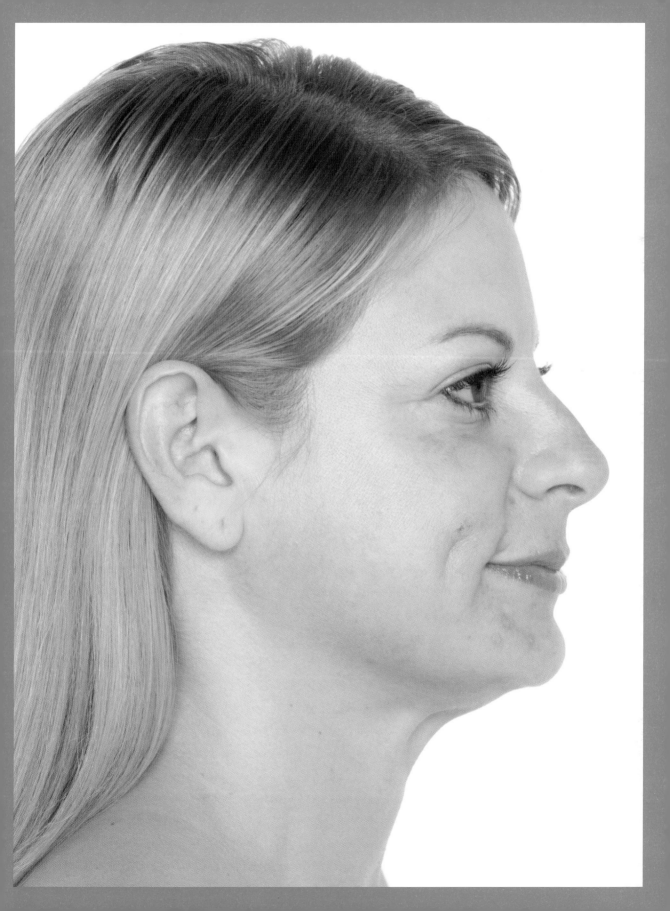

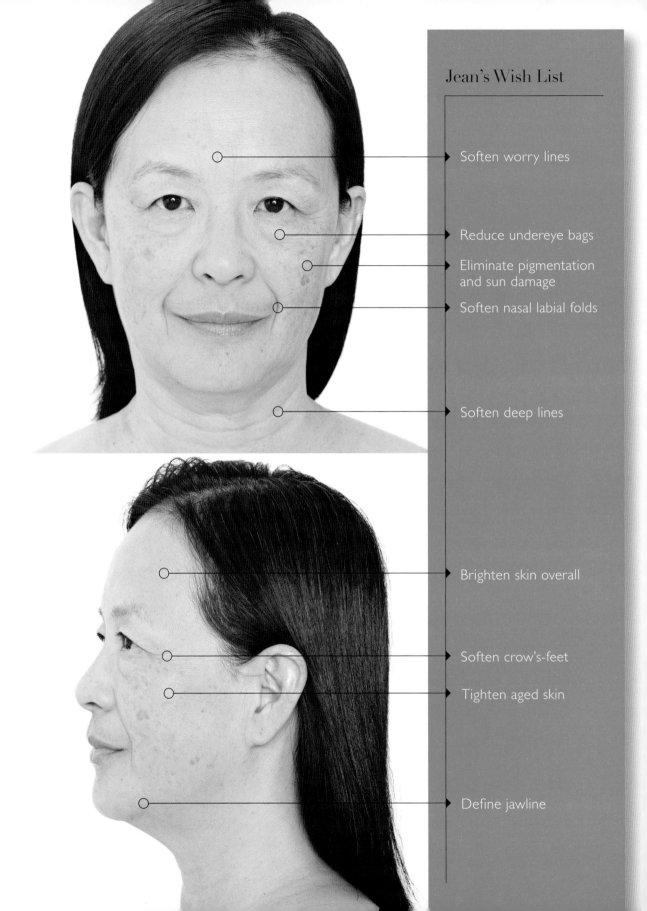

Jean's Wish List

Soften worry lines

Reduce undereye bags

Eliminate pigmentation
and sun damage

Soften nasal labial folds

Soften deep lines

Brighten skin overall

Soften crow's-feet

Tighten aged skin

Define jawline

Anti-aging, pigmentation

Jean is a brand-new grandmother, lives in Southern California, and works as a real-estate agent. When Jean's kids were young, she spent a lot of time in the sun at their soccer and baseball games, and she didn't care for her skin then or even wear sunscreen (although she does now). She has some blotchiness, which started about four years ago as she entered perimenopause. She volunteered for this makeover because she hoped to "learn how to slow down my skin's wrinkling and dryness and clear up some of the pigmentation."

Typical of many women who tend to neglect themselves while taking care of everyone else, Jean said, "I wish I had done this makeover when I was 30 or 40. You shouldn't wait until you're almost 60 to start taking care of your skin, but I'm hoping that it's never too late." She'd noticed that we tend to age faster as time goes on and wanted to learn better skin care so that the next ten years wouldn't progress as quickly. She's a very smart lady.

My Analysis

Jean is in the anti-aging category. But like many women of Asian ethnicity, she has pigmentation problems, too. She's not particularly sensitive, but she is dry. That dryness gets worse if she's stressed, and that makes her skin appear dull.

With a comprehensive program, I planned to clear Jean's hyperpigmentation and plump up some areas with injectables, especially under her eyes. While she was open to that, she opted not to have Botox.

PRODUCTS

Step 1: Cleanse

- Gentle Daily Wash morning and night

Step 2: Exfoliate

- ExfoliKate Intensive Exfoliating Treatment twice a week

- Micro Glycolic Polisher once a week

Step 3: Treat

- Total Vitamin Antioxidant Complex in the morning

- Quench Hydrating Face Serum morning and night

- Refrigerator Cream for the patches of hyperpigmentation

Step 4: Moisturize

- Deep Tissue Repair Cream and Line Release Under Eye Repair Cream morning and night

Step 5: Protect

- Protect SPF 30 Sunscreen

CLINIC TREATMENTS

- Titan®
- Pearl® (two treatments)
- Laser Genesis®
- Radiesse®
- Restylane®

- Juvéderm®
- TCA peel
- Omnilux™ white and red LED lights
- Muscle Lift

DIET AND LIFESTYLE RECOMMENDATIONS

- Reduce diet soda

- Take my Total Vitamin Anti-Aging Supplement

The Results

"My skin has definitely tightened up a lot, and my pores are visibly smaller," Jean said. Most obviously, the injectable fillers plumped up the hollows beneath her eyes, and her dark circles disappeared. However, she had some pigmentation that actually became more pronounced after her second Pearl treatment, so I corrected that with a TCA peel. This is a typical example of how we put together the puzzle: finding out what works for each individual, and what needs reevaluating.

Jean told me that she fell in love with my products, especially the Total Vitamin Antioxidant Complex and the Quench Hydrating Face Serum. She said that she wanted to advise younger women to do as much as they could possibly afford, as early as they can, by budgeting a certain amount for skin care. As she noted, "I look back and think that if I'd done before what I'm doing for myself now, I probably would have much better skin. It's hard to reverse everything, but if you start at 30, you won't need to." Despite being almost twice that age herself, Jean looks amazing!

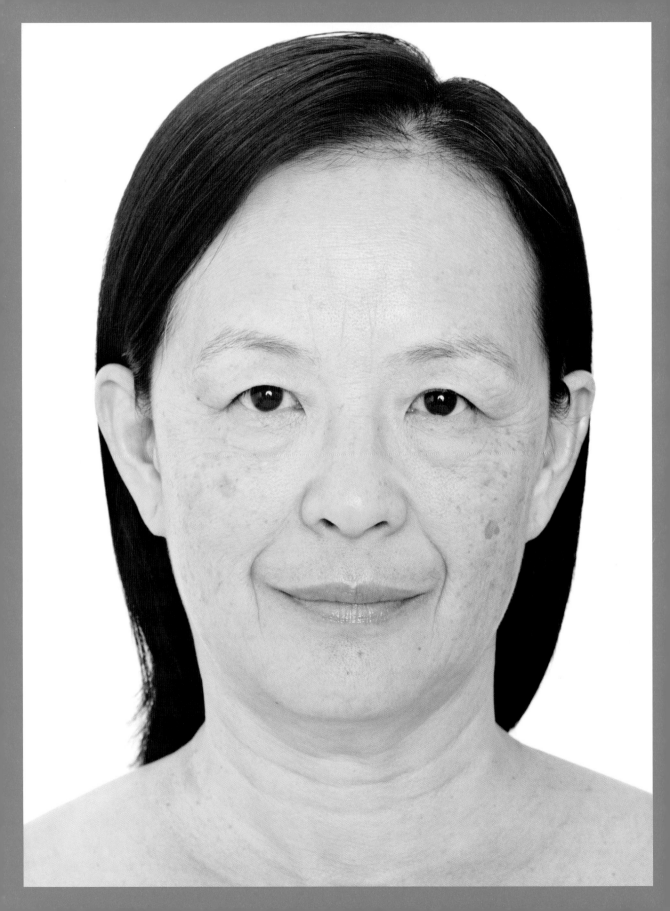

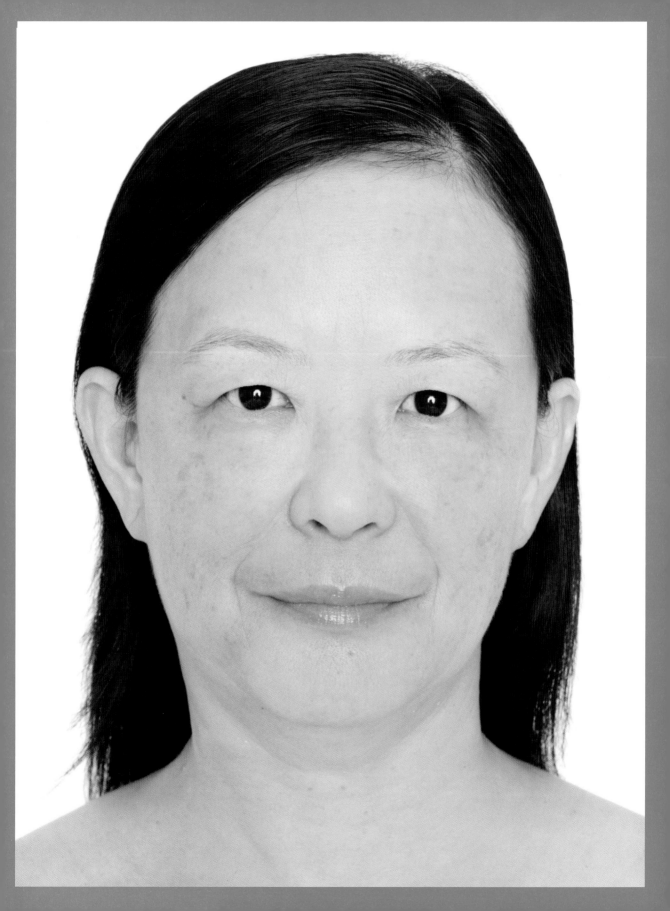

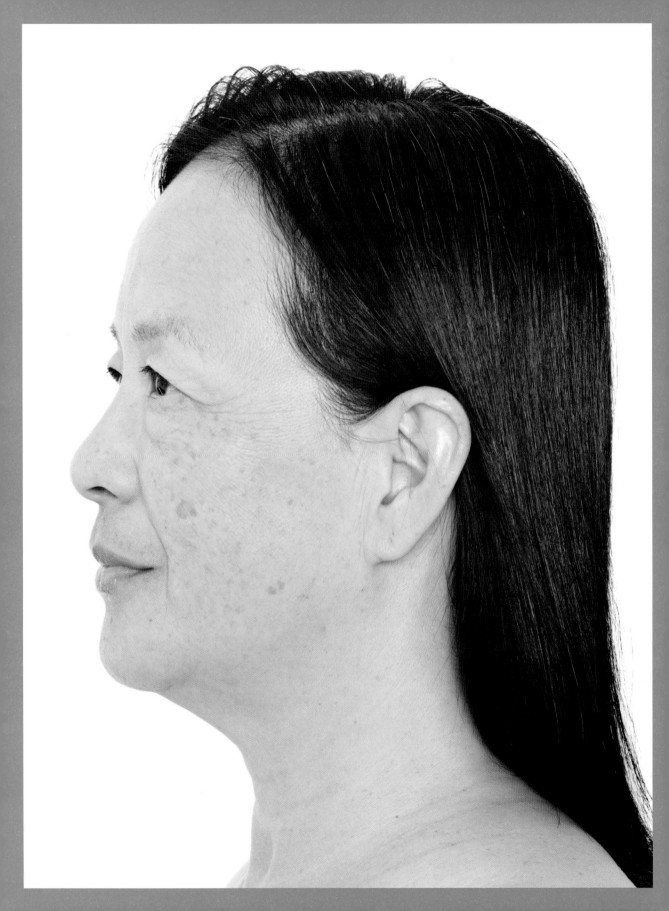

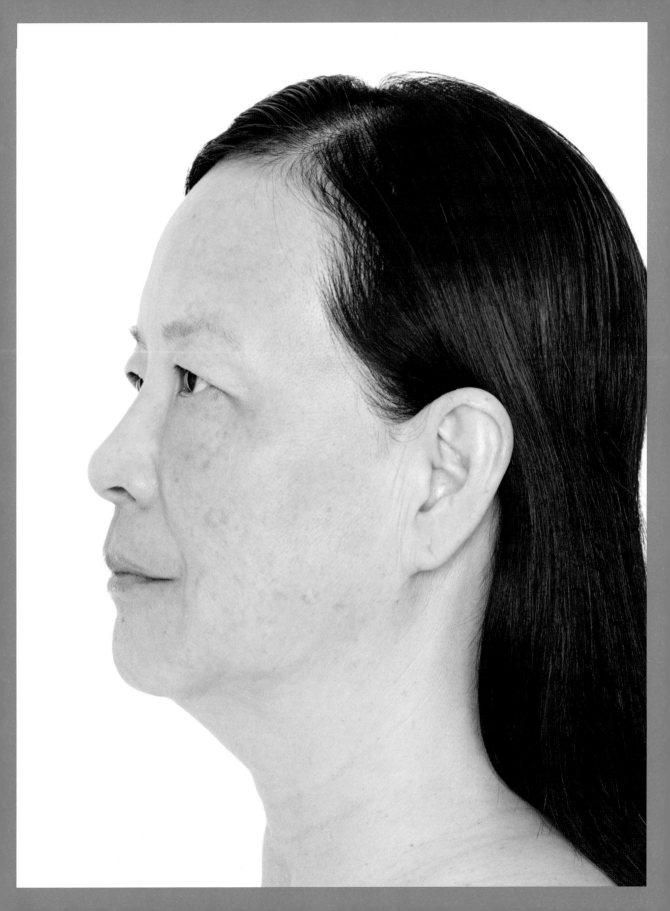

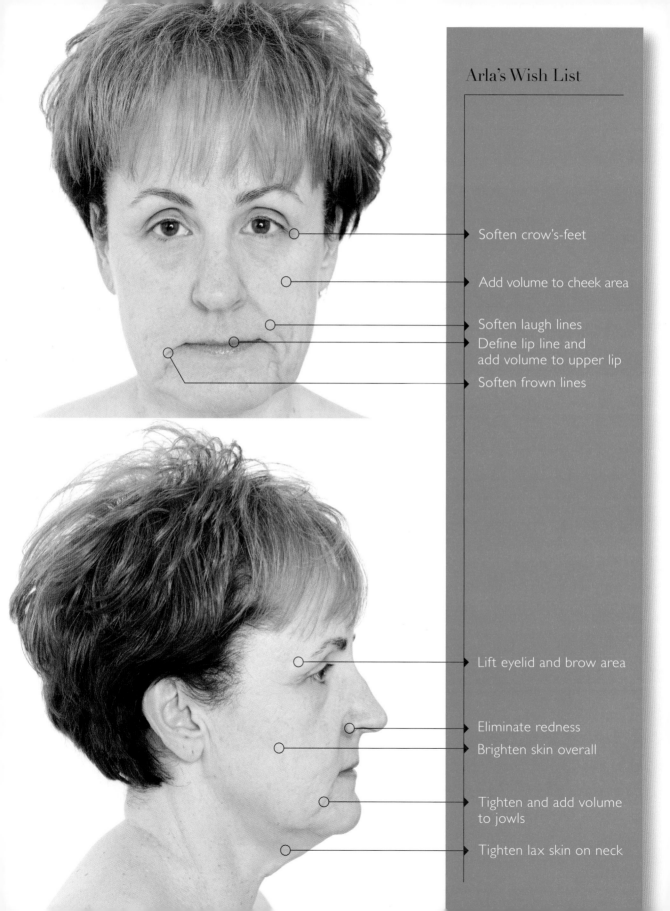

Arla's Wish List

Soften crow's-feet

Add volume to cheek area

Soften laugh lines

Define lip line and
add volume to upper lip

Soften frown lines

Lift eyelid and brow area

Eliminate redness

Brighten skin overall

Tighten and add volume
to jowls

Tighten lax skin on neck

ARLA JORDAN, 52:

Anti-aging, acne scarring

I begged Arla to be a part of this book. She is so youthful, yet her face didn't reflect her vibrant spirit. Although she's really fair, after having heatstroke once as a child, she fortunately got into the habit of staying out of the sun for most of her life. This has served her well, and the effects are obvious—Arla remarkably doesn't have any visible signs of sun damage. However, her skin did exhibit significant laxity, along with some scarring from teenage breakouts.

Arla also mentioned that she wasn't really happy with the way her mouth turned down, and she didn't like her lip because it was "thin and receded" and she could never wear lipstick. Arla has a lot of energy and a caring spirit; she really wanted her face to reflect that.

My Analysis

Arla's main problem was the sagging around her mouth and jawline, so I decided to spot treat her. I believed that she was a perfect candidate for Titan and injectables, which would give her back some of the elasticity and volume she'd lost. She also had deep expression lines, and I knew I'd need to use Botox to soften them up as well. I very naturally added definition and volume to her lip.

PRODUCTS

Step 1: Cleanse

- Gentle Daily Wash morning and night

- Purify Exfoliating Cleanser at night

Step 2: Exfoliate

- ExfoliKate Intensive Exfoliating Treatment twice a week

Step 3: Treat

- Total Vitamin Antioxidant Complex and Quench Hydrating Face Serum morning and night

Step 4: Moisturize

- Nourish Daily Moisture in the morning

- Deep Tissue Repair Cream at night

- Line Release Under Eye Repair Cream morning and night

Step 5: Protect

- Protect SPF 30 Sunscreen

CLINIC TREATMENTS

- Laser Genesis®
- Titan®
- Pearl®
- Botox®

- Juvéderm®
- Radiesse®
- Omnilux™ white LED light
- Muscle Lift

DIET AND LIFESTYLE RECOMMENDATIONS

- Watch white-sugar intake

- Try to stay away from coffee (which Arla liked to sip all day), as it's dehydrating and will slow down healing. Switch to green tea for the antioxidants.

- Take my Total Vitamin Anti-Aging Supplement

The Results

Here's what Arla said: "I was somewhat hesitant about having the injectables and Botox, but now that I've had it done, I would line up to do it again and again and again! They make a difference in what people see as your demeanor, but they don't distort your features."

Arla's was a pretty challenging case because of the weight of her laxity. However, the results really improved the areas that bothered her most—that is, her lips and the corners of her mouth—and the tone and texture of her skin is now incredibly refined. Overall, Arla's face looks naturally fuller, softer, and younger. "I've actually had people I don't even know comment on how nice my skin is," she told me. "I've never felt so good about myself."

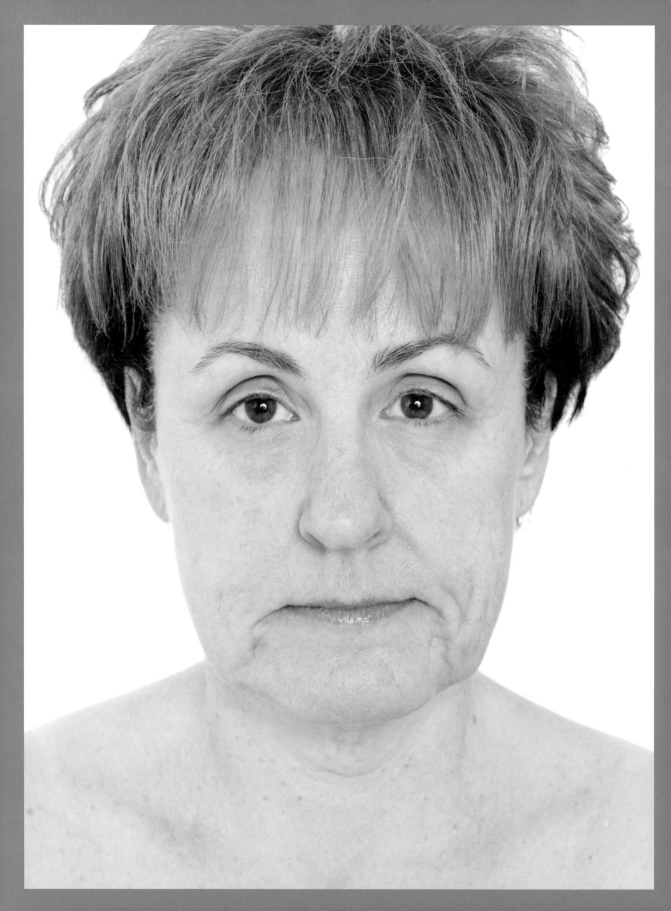

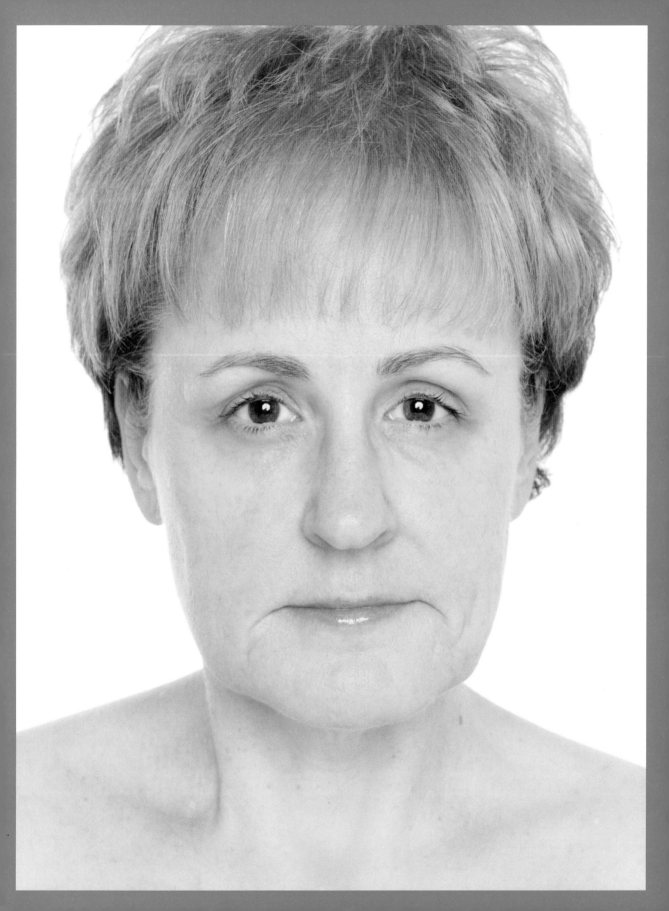

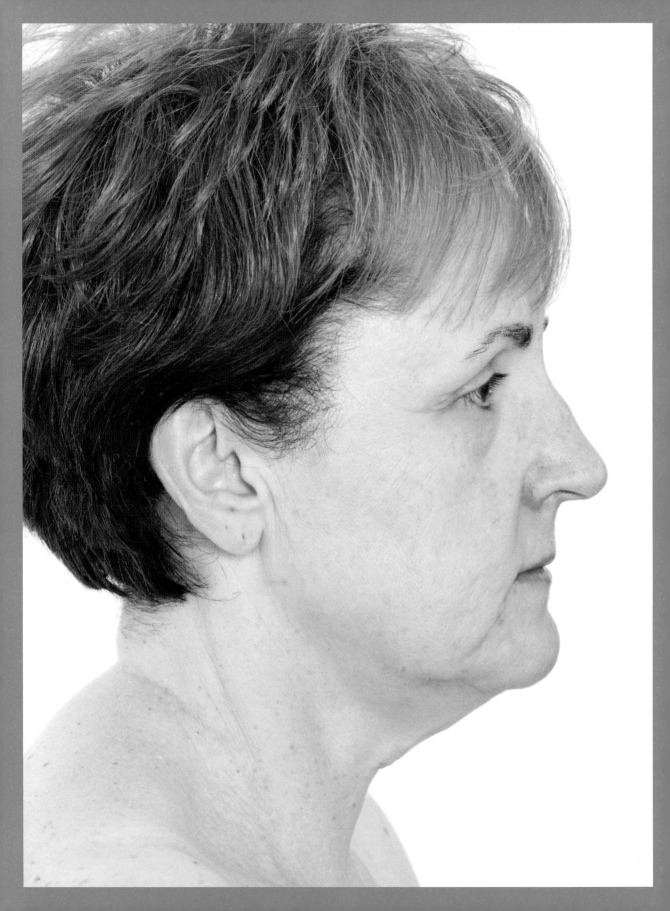

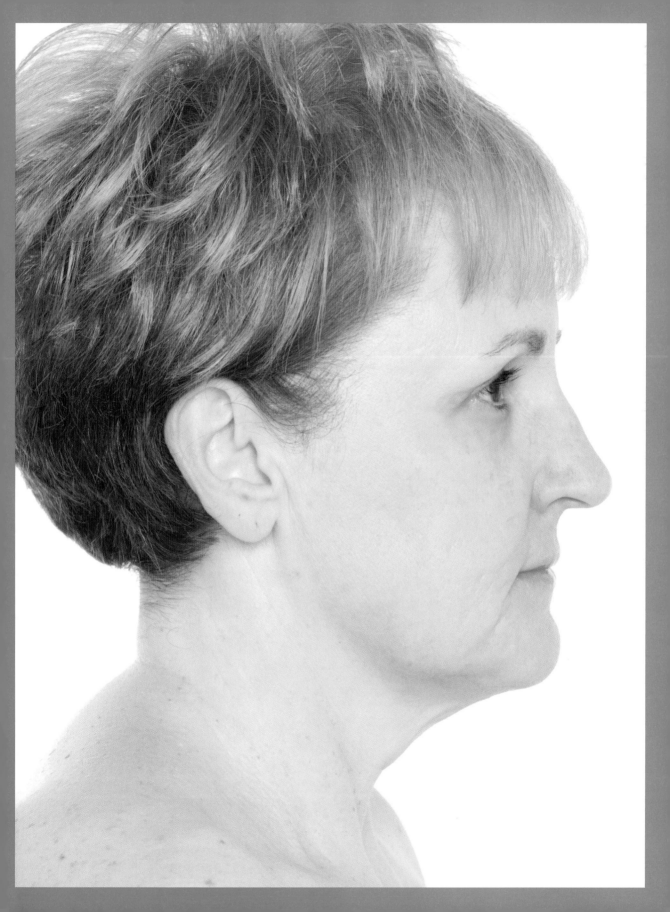

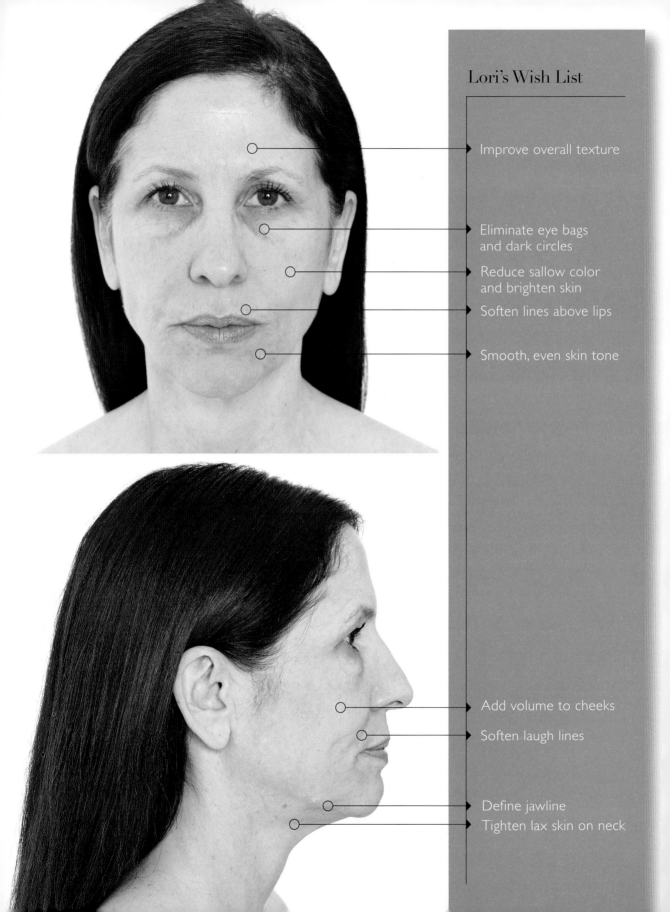

Lori's Wish List

Improve overall texture

Eliminate eye bags
and dark circles

Reduce sallow color
and brighten skin

Soften lines above lips

Smooth, even skin tone

Add volume to cheeks

Soften laugh lines

Define jawline

Tighten lax skin on neck

Anti-aging

Lori is a singer-songwriter and actress, so looking her best and appearing youthful is important to her. She's also a devotee of a practice called siddha yoga, which is not a physical pursuit, but rather a spiritual form of meditation. "My troubles are answered and I can control my mind when I meditate, and then I feel better in general," she told me. She's already a client of mine, and while her sense of inner peace was inspiring, I thought there were a few things we could still do for her exterior self.

My Analysis

My team and I had done a lot of work on Lori's skin already. Even so, she had some lines around her lips from smoking and dehydration, expression lines and folds that could be softened with injectables, and a bit of discoloration around her eyes. My plan was to "polish" her up and make her skin milky beautiful.

PRODUCTS

Step 1: Cleanse

- Gentle Daily Wash morning and night

Step 2: Exfoliate

- ExfoliKate Intensive Exfoliating Treatment twice a week

Step 3: Treat

- Total Vitamin Antioxidant Complex and Quench Hydrating Face Serum morning and night

Step 4: Moisturize

- Deep Tissue Repair Cream and Line Release Under Eye Repair Cream morning and night

Step 5: Protect

- Protect SPF 30 Sunscreen

CLINIC TREATMENTS

- Titan®
- Laser Genesis®
- Pearl®
- Botox®

- Radiesse®
- Restylane®
- Juvéderm®
- Omnilux™ white and red LED lights

■ Take my Total Vitamin Anti-Aging Supplement

The Results

Lori's skin is as close to perfect as it's possible to be. The bags under her eyes are gone, and her complexion is flawless. Of course she had quite good skin to start with, and she was often taken for younger than her almost-50 years. But now people are guessing that she's in her early 30s! That just goes to show that you don't need to have major issues to see a vast improvement in your skin.

"It was the best experience of my life, and I feel like a queen!" Lori exclaimed. "This has changed me not just physically but also mentally. I feel so good about myself that my attitude has become lighter and friendlier, and other people are responding to it. I believe this has set me off on a new course in life. I actually cried the last day of my treatments."

Hearing Lori's story made *me* cry, too. It's so amazing to watch the physical changes in someone, and then feel his or her personal transformation all the way down to your heart.

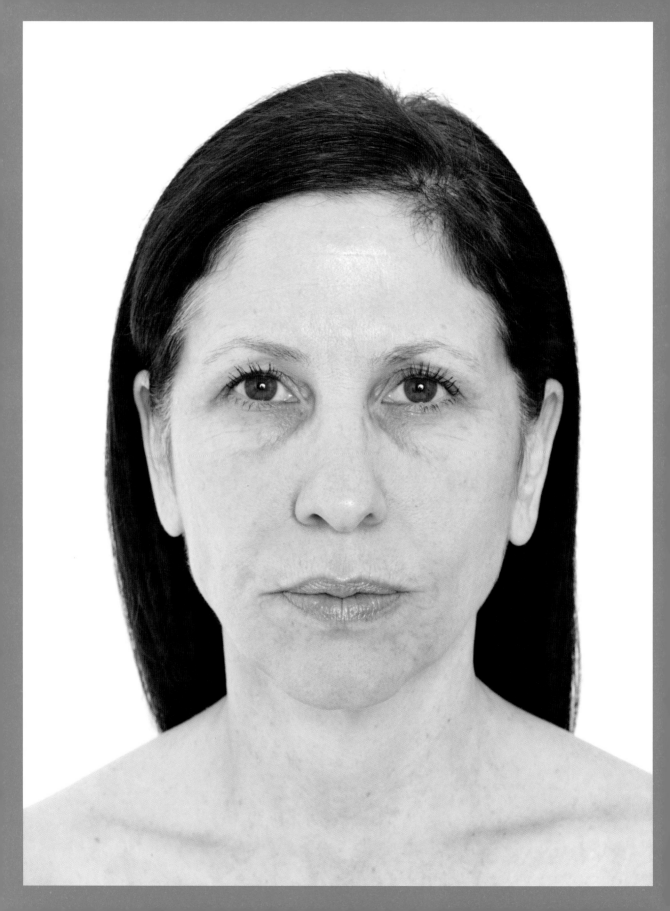

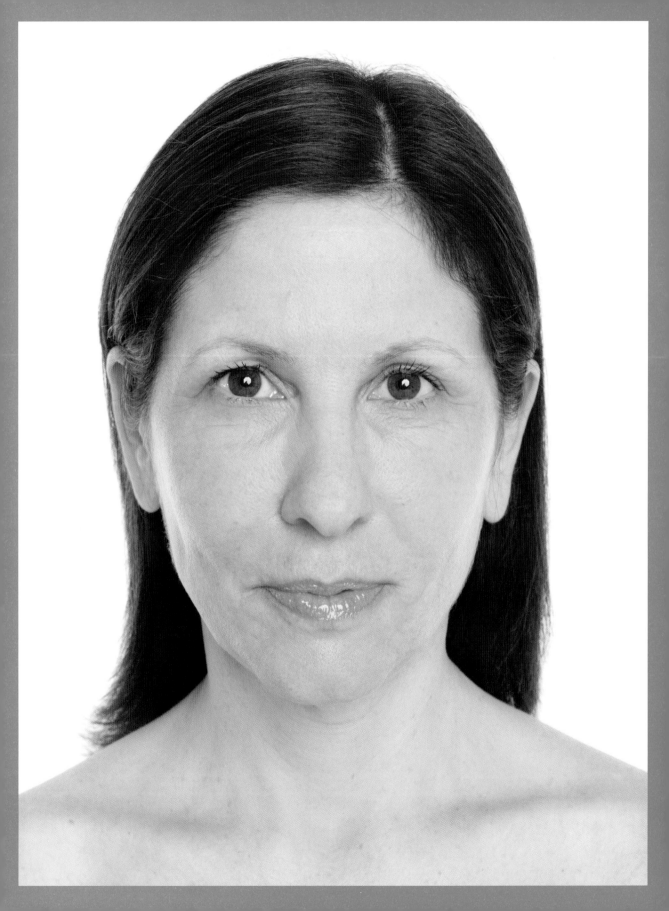

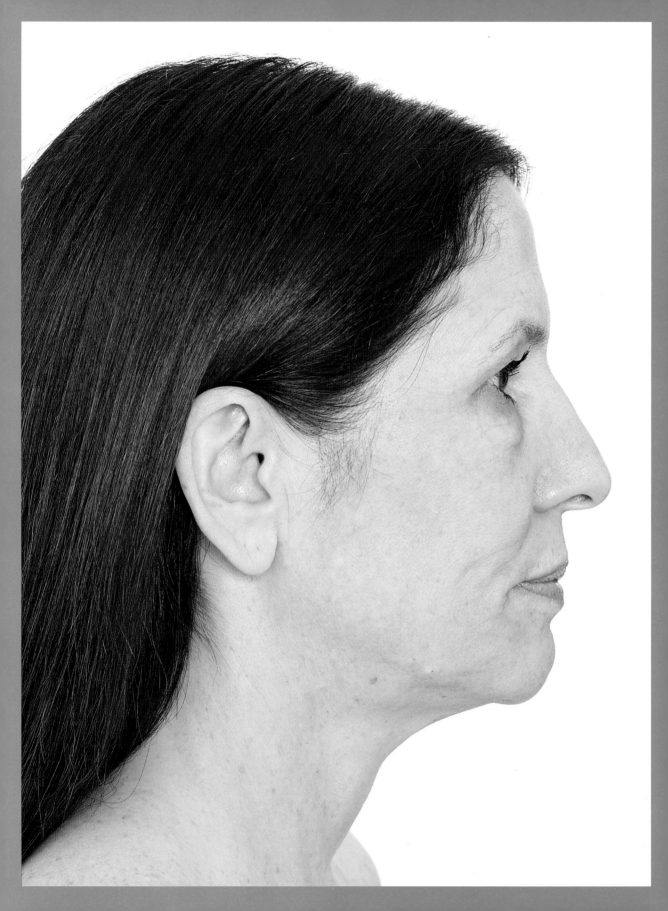

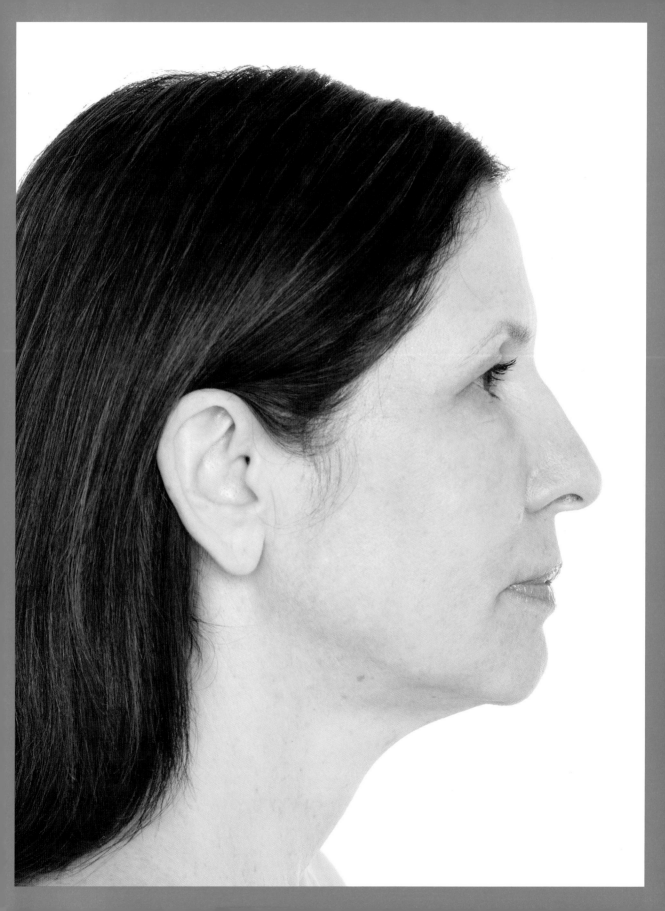

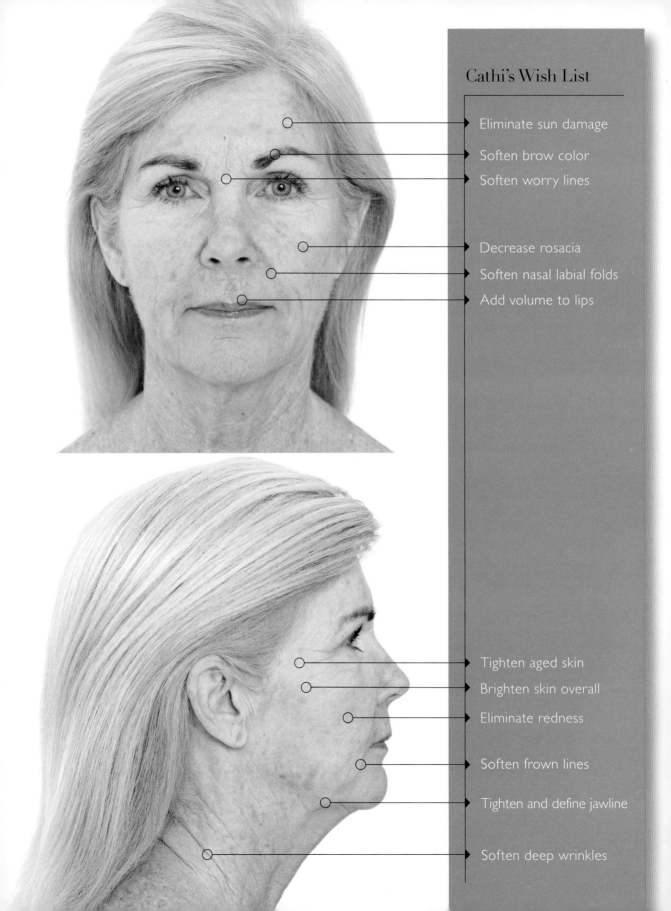

Cathi's Wish List

Eliminate sun damage

Soften brow color

Soften worry lines

Decrease rosacia

Soften nasal labial folds

Add volume to lips

Tighten aged skin

Brighten skin overall

Eliminate redness

Soften frown lines

Tighten and define jawline

Soften deep wrinkles

CATHI MYERS, 62:

Sun damage, anti-aging, precancerous spots

Cathi is a California girl, born and bred, who lived on the beach as a teenager. She confessed to lying out in the sun slathered in baby oil and cocoa butter, in search of the perfect tan. I'm sure that many people her age can identify with that! She never really stopped being a lover of the outdoors all through her adulthood—she still goes to the beach, walks, plays tennis, and rides motorcycles. And she told me that her biggest accomplishment in life is raising four now-grown kids.

Cathi acknowledged that she didn't take care of her skin until she was in her 30s, at which point she just started using moisturizers. Now, thankfully, she's aware of the importance of sunscreen, since she's had pre-melanomas removed from her back. Even so, when she came in for a facial, we spotted something on her nose that we recommended she have checked out. It turned out to be a basal cell carcinoma, which was taken off.

"I don't use much makeup," Cathi said, "just some mineral powder." She told me that she'd like to look more like the way she feels, which is a common theme I've heard with my clients. So I vowed to make that happen.

My Analysis

Boy, oh boy, did Cathi have some serious sun damage! This included visible actinic keratoses (growths on the skin caused by sun exposure) as well as splotches and patches of discoloration all over her face, neck, and chest. Cathi represents so many women who have this type of skin, especially in the "Sunbelt" states of California, Arizona, Texas, and Florida. It's better to prevent this kind of damage, but it can also be reversed with lasers and a little patience.

Since Cathi also tended to be sensitive and prone to redness and irritation, I had her go through what I call a full "3-D," or three-dimensional treatment. Basically, that means that we worked on every single level of her skin. In addition, I specifically instructed her to use all of the products I gave her, all the way down her neck and chest.

PRODUCTS

Step 1: Cleanse

- Gentle Daily Wash morning and night

Step 2: Exfoliate

- ExfoliKate Intensive Exfoliating Treatment twice a week. My team and I did warn Cathi that wherever she had those keratoses, the spots would get "angry," but it was okay because we were helping slough them off.

Step 3: Treat

- Total Vitamin Antioxidant Complex and Quench Hydrating Face Serum morning and night

- Refrigerator Cream three times a week, at night, for a couple of months

Step 4: Moisturize

- Deep Tissue Repair Cream and Line Release Under Eye Repair cream morning and night

Step 5: Protect

- Protect SPF 55 Serum Sunscreen

CLINIC TREATMENTS

- Omnilux™ white and red LED lights
- Titan® (three treatments)
- Laser Genesis®
- Pearl®

- IPL on her face, chest, and hands
- Botox®
- Juvéderm®
- Radiesse®

DIET AND LIFESTYLE RECOMMENDATION

- Take my Total Vitamin Anti-Aging Supplement

The Results

At the end of the process, Cathi announced, "I feel unbelievable! So good, in fact, that I don't wear any makeup, although I *never* go out without sunscreen anymore."

Not only did we eliminate so many signs of sun damage from this wonderful woman's face and down her chest, we also lightened up her old scars from having the precancerous spots removed and refined her pores. "Everyone notices and comments," Cathi said. "I couldn't be happier with the experience; it was the best thing I have ever done for myself." And after her daughter sent some pictures to Cathi's grandchildren, she proudly said, "Even my grandkids could tell!"

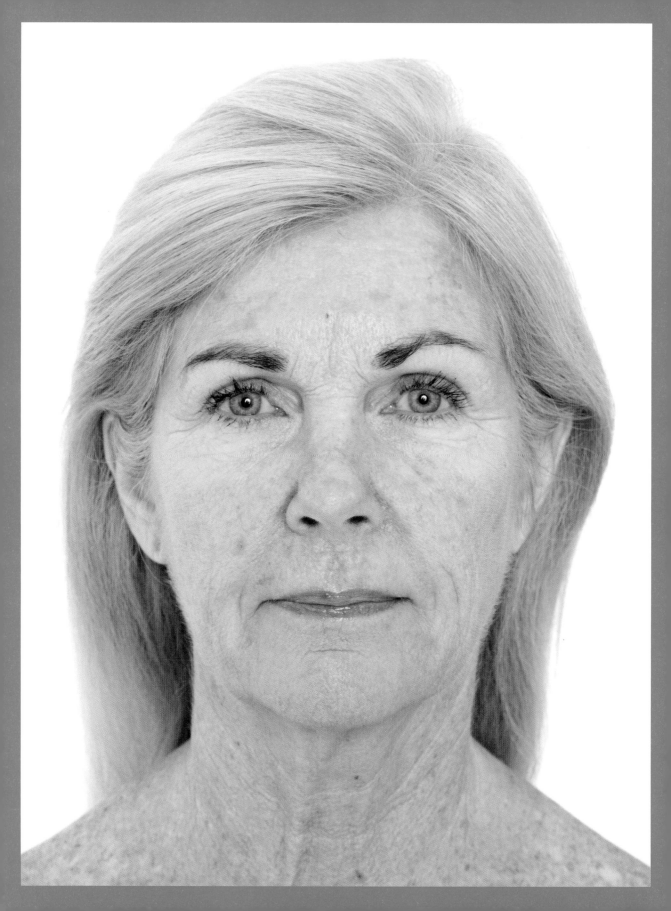

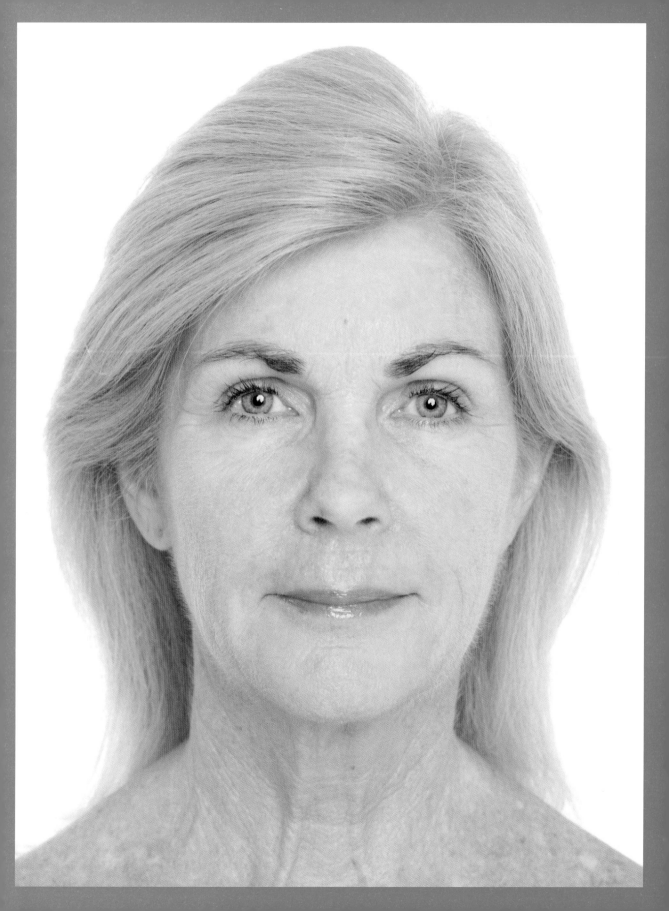

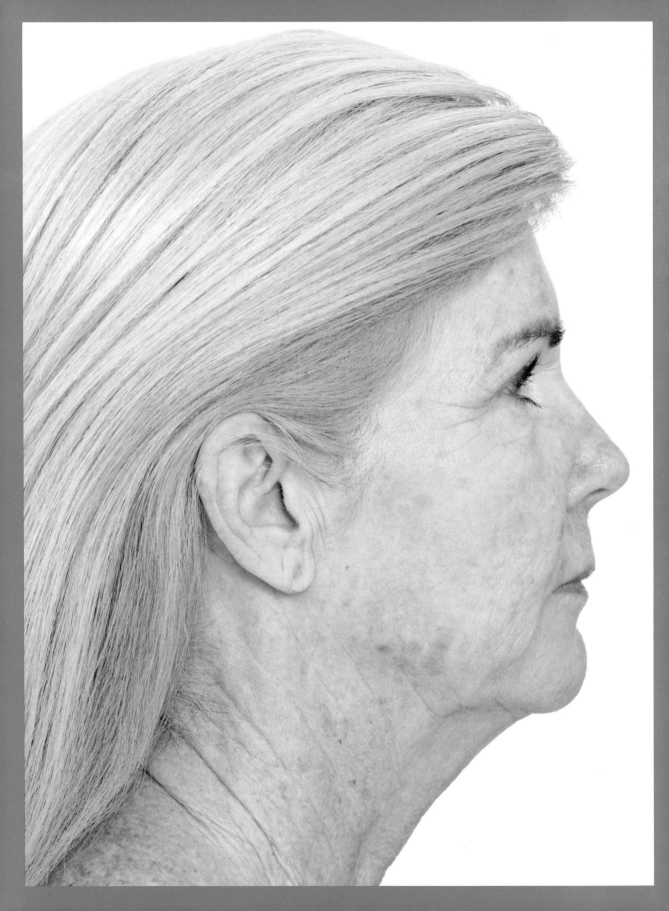

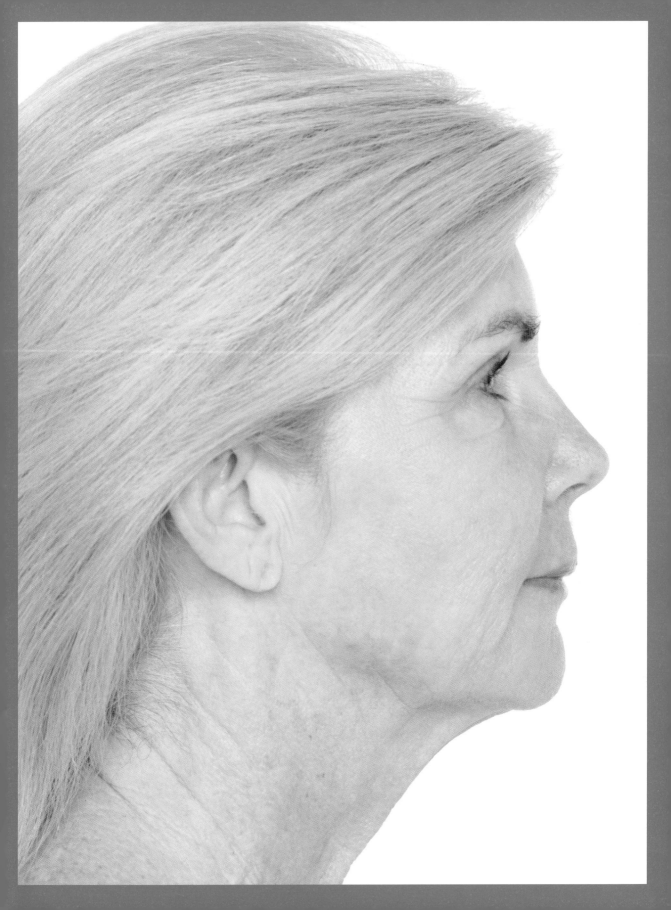

MY TEAM: THE SKIN HEALTH EXPERTS

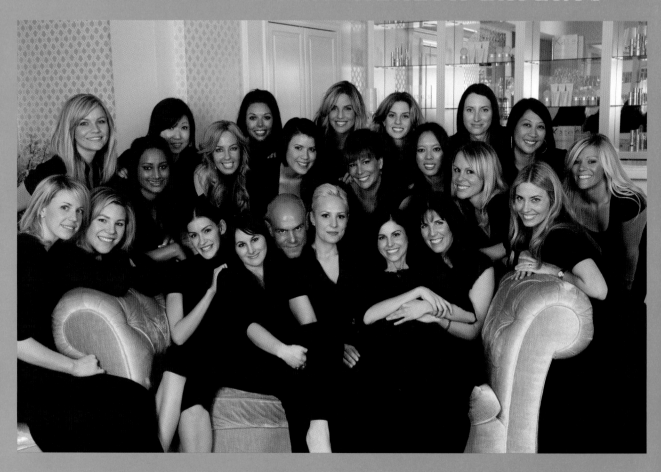

Transforming the skin of these clients was a team effort. The RNs, estheticians, clinic staff, and the rest of my team dedicated hundreds of hours to this cause. They worked unbelievably hard executing the treatments, strategies, and programs. These are the most talented and dedicated professionals in the business, and together we share the same passion, the same goals, and the same professional motto: "changing skin, changing lives." And we do it every day!

Transformations can take place at any age, on any skin type, which I believe the makeovers in this chapter demonstrate. Next up, I discuss specific advice for certain phases and decades of life. Knowing these things, and then applying them, can help keep your skin on track, whatever stage you happen to be in.

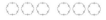

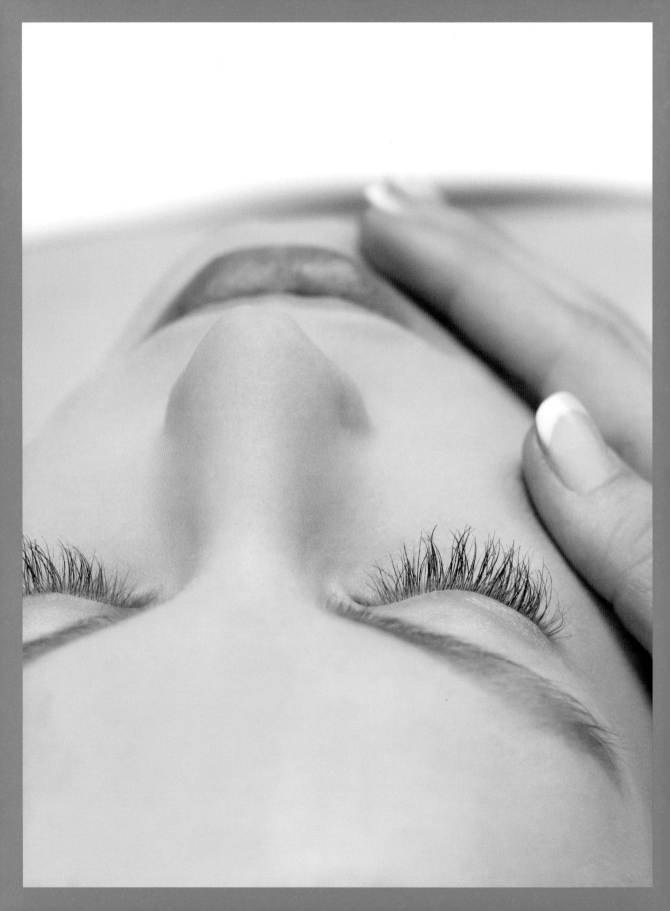

PART IV

Complexion Affection!

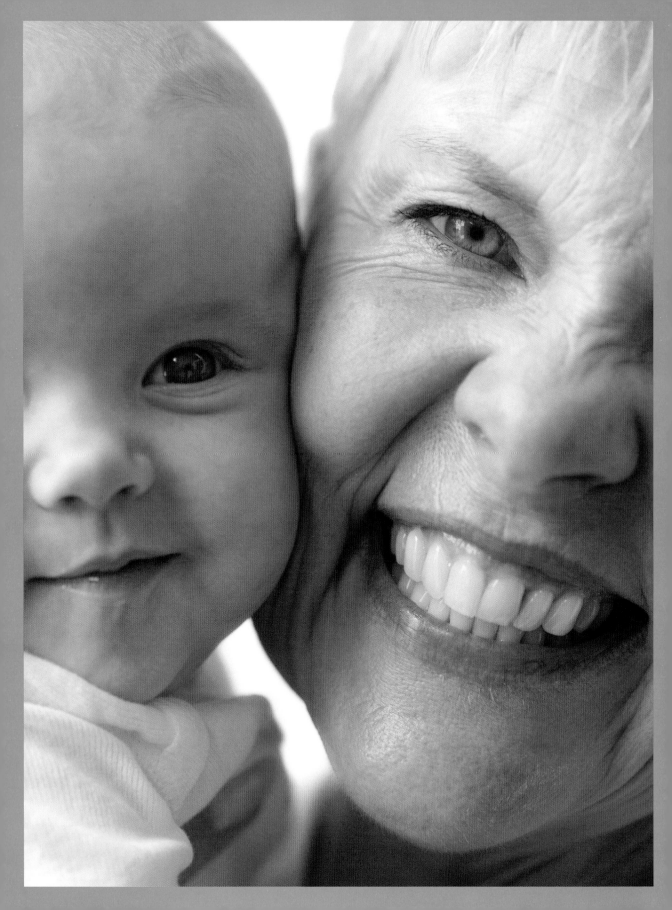

CHAPTER 10

Stages of Skin Health

Our skin is called our "birthday suit" for a reason. We're born in it, and we wear it our whole lives. Wouldn't it be great if it stayed the same as it was when we were babies: soft, silky, plumped up with moisture, unwrinkled, unblemished, and undamaged by the environment? It sure would, but unfortunately, that doesn't happen. Instead, our skin becomes a little more timeworn with each passing year. The freckles on our forearms and the crow's-feet on our faces are the tattoos of life—not the kind we ask for,

but the kind we do pay for.

When my clinic team and I were talking to our makeover subjects from Part III, we heard one thing over and over. While their words may have been different, the message was the same: "I wish I'd started taking care of my skin earlier instead of playing catch-up now." But you know what, most of us didn't know any better.

Happily, in the last 20 years or so, we've become much more aware of the damage various unhealthy habits such as suntanning, smoking, eating poorly, and simple neglect can do to our complexion. Education, science, and improved products have all contributed toward our taking better care of our skin at earlier ages. But even though we're savvier, I still worry that not everyone is translating the knowledge into action. For every young person who's compliant about putting on sunscreen every day or who meticulously cleanses morning and night, I hear another saying, "Well, I know I should, but . . ."

I can tell you that my Skin Health Pyramid applies *throughout* life, and it's important that you know how to treat your skin at various stages. As your skin changes, so should your regimen and your treatment menu. What you need in your 20s is very different from what you need in your 50s.

Here is some specific advice on how to take care of your skin throughout the decades and major phases of life. But remember the most important thing: you have to continuously give it love!

Childhood

There's no better place to start than at the beginning—with that precious baby skin we all envy. Diaper rash is, of course, the first skin problem we usually have to deal with. Here are some tips for avoiding it:

- Let your baby go "commando" for a while every day to air out that area that's usually encased in a diaper.

- Change your little one as soon as she wets or soils her diaper. Dampness and ammonia from the urine can contribute to the condition.

- Wash your baby's bottom during every change. Use plain warm water, or a mild soap if soiled, and rinse well so that no soap residue is left.

- Gently pat her bottom dry: rubbing can be irritating. (Think of how irritated your nose gets when you have a cold.)

- Don't use plastic pants over diapers because they can create a hot, damp environment.

Even when you take precautions, diaper rash happens. I know this very well, since my son had a pretty bad case of it at one point. I tried over-the-counter medications and found one product from Germany—Penaten Creme—that really helped him. It's basically zinc oxide, which is a barrier and a healer as well. However, you have to be careful if you're using zinc products because they can also dry the skin a bit. If you moisturize first and then apply the zinc, you'll be good to go.

Small children can have more significant skin conditions, too. Eczema, for instance, is a growing problem among American kids and can be hereditary. (Mine started in childhood, and I was so worried when I had my baby—happily, he didn't get my skin.) Eczema is an allergic reaction, and you need to learn what the triggers are. They might be food or external things such as soaps, dust, fabrics, and so forth. Stress can also contribute if you're prone to the condition, and this even applies to children.

Eczema is sometimes confused with psoriasis, which is less common in very young children. Psoriasis is not allergy related—it's an immune-system malfunction where skin cells reproduce too quickly and pile up in patches on the surface of the skin. For both of these problems, I believe in really hydrating and moisturizing the affected areas. Some doctors say not to take a lot of baths, but I'm with the ones who think the opposite. I believe that the individual should be in water more, for hydration purposes, and then immediately put on a moisturizer to seal the water in. I'm a huge proponent of Curél brand moisturizer and use it myself, as it really soothes the skin.

To make baths even more comforting, try putting in colloidal oatmeal (that simply means oatmeal that's ground fine enough to disperse through the water and not sink into sludge at the bottom). You can make it yourself: grind about ⅓ cup of rolled oats to a fine powder in a food processor or coffee grinder, and stir it into a warm bath, which you let your little one soak in for 10 to 15 minutes.

Such a bath can also be helpful if your infant is suffering from "baby acne," which can be the result of the mother's diet when breast-feeding. Keep in mind that your little boy or girl has an undeveloped digestive system and can be sensitive or even allergic to things that you as a mother are not, and you need to pay special attention to your diet when breast-feeding. I've found that eating a lot of dairy products can, for some babies, contribute to various skin allergies and other discomforts.

The golden rule for childhood skin care is this: *Less is more.* That applies to everything. You don't want to put a lot of chemicals on kids, and you also want to be careful with natural products, too. Note that "natural" doesn't necessarily translate to "harmless," and certain remedies such as essential oils can really inflame a baby's skin.

Teens

Breakouts are happening; kids at school are mean; proms and first dates are being ruined by giant zits; there's a lot of drama and crying. Welcome to the teen years, which can be *devastating* for the boys and girls going through them.

Blemishes and all of the angst that accompanies them are, of course, mainly a result of hormones changing. There are some fortunate ones who don't get acne because it does also have a genetic component—if one or both of the parents had it, then the kids are predisposed, too. Yet boys are especially prone to acne, because testosterone is the main culprit. When the body starts pumping out this male hormone (and girls have it, too, in lesser amounts), it also stimulates the skin's oil glands to go crazy producing sebum. The excess oil blocks pores, and the next thing you know, you have acne, blackheads, whiteheads, and inflammation.

At this stage of life, you really don't want to mess with hormones. I also don't recommend going with Retin-A or other harsh topical products. You may be successful in drying up the oil, but you're also likely to cause a lot of surface irritation. And with that much irritation, you need to wear sunscreen, and this age group just cannot be relied upon to do that.

I'm not a big proponent of the prescription drug Accutane, except in one very specific instance: if you're dealing with severe cystic acne that will leave a lifetime of scarring, then it might be the way to go. You need to know that there are some measures we skin-care professionals can take to deal with the scarring later, but it's better to avoid getting it in the first place.

So what do I recommend for teenage acne? I have a three-point plan for dealing with it:

1. Light treatments. This is where the blue and red light series (LED treatments) are absolutely amazing. The lights are safe, don't involve drugs, don't require the kids to do anything other than show up, and are really effective.

2. A simple skin-care regimen. Boys are tough because they often resist this step. Usually, though, I can get them on three products: a cleanser and an exfoliant to use in the shower, and then some timed-release benzoyl peroxide. If they really care about their skin, I'll put them on a kaolin (clay) mask, too. Girls are usually more into all of this, and they're much more compliant about using products.

3. Lifestyle changes. Exercise promotes oxygen and blood flow to the skin, and that encourages healthy cells. It also helps regulate the endocrine system, which produces those hormones. In addition, physical activity discharges stress, and playing sports can boost confidence lost from having a face full of acne. Sweating can be instrumental in cleaning out pores, but only if individuals are also meticulous about cleanliness. For example, lots of boys get sweaty and dirty and exposed to bacteria, and some I've met don't even take a shower right away. I still have to tell my husband to get in the shower after a long tennis match. *Seriously!*

Skin-telligence:

BY THE HAIR ON YOUR CHINNY-CHIN-CHIN!
This isn't exactly the sexiest subject, but ladies, it's a sad fact that as we get older, hair on the face tends to crop up along the jaw or on the chin. So unless you want to grow these guys out and wear them in a braid, here's my advice.

You can pluck the hair out, but that can cause injury to the follicle, resulting in a blemish, bump, postpluck infection, or scar. If you do pluck, always dab a little witch hazel or tea-tree oil on the spot afterward. Electrolysis works, but it usually takes a lot of visits and is less effective than laser hair removal. If you opt for laser hair removal, be sure not to pluck for at least four to six weeks prior to your appointment. You'll probably have to do three to six treatments, or even more, depending on how dark your skin is and how stubborn the hairs are. And because hormones are constantly in flux, they may come back.

Please note that an unusual amount of hair growth on your face can be the result of a condition known as polycystic ovary syndrome. If you think that this might be the case, consult your doctor and ask her to test your hormones.

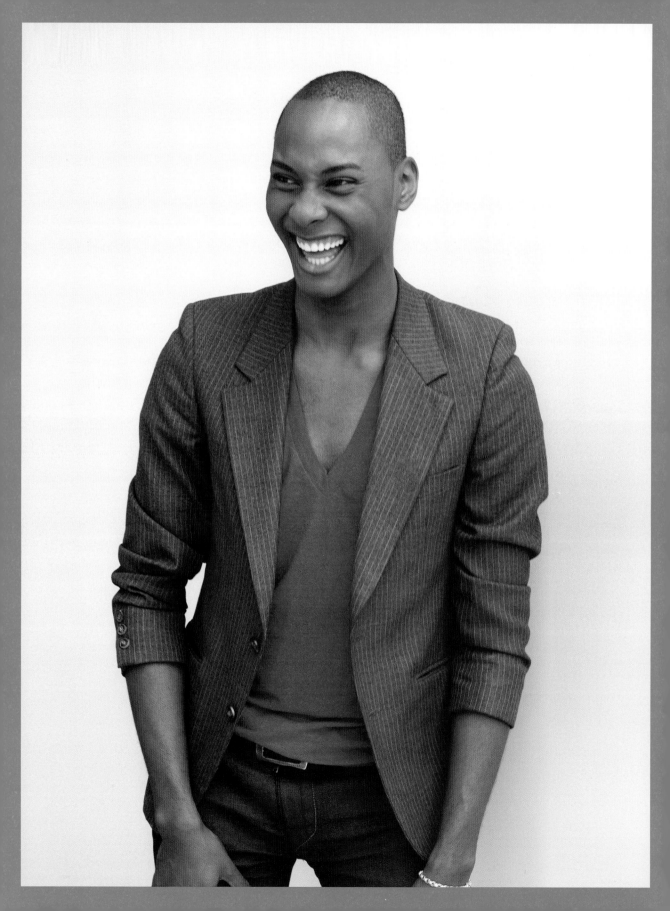

ANDREW PETTIT: MY STORY

I've struggled with my skin since I was young: I first started breaking out when I was about 12 or 13. I was embarrassed, self-conscious, and incredibly insecure. I don't have a really good "before" picture (before Kate, that is!), because I pretty much refused to be in photos. (The photos below should make you understand why I felt this way.) So there's a lot of my life that is missing in photos.

I had severe cystic acne and was so frustrated; I tried everything. Doctors put me on antibiotics, and at first that helped—but as soon as I'd go off of them, my skin would go back to how it had been before or even get worse. Over time, they just didn't work at all. The drugs made me feel really sick, too. I wanted healthy skin, but I didn't want to risk my overall health for it. My breakouts got so bad there wasn't a spot on my face where there wasn't acne. Nothing was working, and I felt terrible.

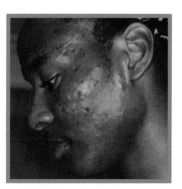

I love music, and I've been singing gospel and R & B since I was three. I

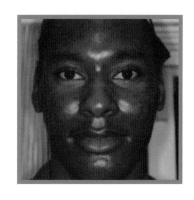

can't tell you how hard it was for me to get up onstage when I was breaking out and not feeling good about myself. It was almost impossible. As a singer, a lot of my life consists of shows, photo shoots, and different engagements in front of people. So on top of worrying about how I'm going to perform or how well I'll sing, I had to deal with fears about how I look.

I first heard about Kate while watching a TV special on Hollywood beauty secrets. I was glued to the screen because of my own struggle with my skin. She seemed different, so I figured I'd give her program a try. Kate and the girls at the clinic took me under their wing and truly cared about me. They said that I was one of the most challenging cases they had ever seen, but they weren't going to give up until I was clear. So I did a lot of treatments: the facials helped clean out my skin, the red and blue LED lights got rid of the breakouts, and the Laser Genesis and the Titan improved the scarring and discoloration.

It took about a year of work, but now my skin is clear. Really clear. Like baby's-butt clear! It is *so* smooth, and there aren't any painful blemishes. This has seriously changed my life and the way I feel about myself. A few months ago I was walking down the street, and a modeling agent approached me. I couldn't believe it! I never could have imagined just how amazing clear skin would make me feel.

For me, the most incredible thing is that I don't have to worry about my skin anymore. I'm free to concentrate on something higher, which I believe is my calling: my music. All that energy I used to spend feeling down and worrying about my skin is now spent on something positive. When I walk onstage now and get under those lights, I feel confident and don't even think about my skin. I think about my love of music, performance, and connecting with the audience.

Whenever I step into Kate Somerville's clinic, it's like a second home to me. I love everyone there . . . they make me feel (and look!) so good. I am so happy and grateful to Kate for changing my life. And if I can say one thing to those struggling with skin issues, it's that you really can have beautiful skin. Sometimes it takes work, but it's so possible. Thanks, Kate!

Andrew is an amazing musician and has the heart and the voice of an angel. If you want to hear his music, please check him out: **www.myspace.com/andrewpettitmusic**.

20s

When you're in your early 20s, you can have really good skin. In a best-case scenario, your hormones are settling down; your skin's producing just enough sebum to keep you hydrated; and your cells are turning over quite fast, which keeps your skin looking fresh. This is the time you need to develop an effective basic program to preserve your skin. All you really need to maintain a glowing complexion is a good cleanser, an exfoliant, a moisturizer, and sunscreen.

On the other hand, there are a lot of variables during this phase. You could still have some hormonal upheaval, for instance, or you might go on birth control pills that can affect your skin for better or for worse. I also typically see women having combination skin at this age. So if you're like this and have breakouts in your oily zones, I reiterate what I've said several times before: use acne products *only* where you need them, and be sure to avoid the eye area.

As you hit your late 20s, you might start to see the beginnings of fine lines, and this is the time to start adding in anti-aging products—you want moisturizers and treatments with peptides like Matrixyl. You can start using eye cream, too.

I'd recommend getting facials once a month or every other month at this point. If you want to get into treatments, red and white LED lights will help preserve your skin. Also, get in the habit now of examining your skin regularly for any signs of skin cancer. Melanoma, the most deadly type, tends to hit young people.

When it comes to your lifestyle, you probably need to watch what you eat, since these can often be the "fast food" years. You might be living on your own for the first time and spending long hours establishing yourself in a career or having babies (maybe both). Meals can become a matter of convenience, and your intake of greasy, hormone-laden food is at a maximum. Stress can be a factor, too. Trust me—you'll see the results of all of this reflected in your skin. Establishing healthy habits now will last you a lifetime.

30s

Your cell turnover starts to slow down now, and the surface of your skin can become drier and duller and show signs of sun damage. Keep up with your cleanse/exfoliate/treat/moisturize/protect regimen and regular facials.

This is when you need to start focusing on anti-aging. If you haven't started using peptides already, now is definitely the time to do so, as collagen begins to decrease.

You'll also benefit from using a retinol product or Retin-A. Muscle mass also begins to decline, so microcurrent treatments are effective in combating this. You can bump up to more advanced treatments, too: for example, Laser Genesis will keep fine lines and wrinkles at bay.

In your late 30s, if you have textural issues such as enlarged pores and sun damage, you can start on the Pearl laser and IPL. The use of gentle peels with lactic or glycolic acids can also help reduce the appearance of pore size and smooth out textural issues.

I know what I'm about to say next is controversial, but I think that this is the time to look into Botox *if* you're developing expression lines. People with expressionless faces can remain unlined in their 40s, but when you have an animated face, you can be creating expression lines in your 20s that show up in your 30s and beyond. I'm talking about things like frown lines and vertical lines around your mouth. Using Botox is not a matter of age; when used artfully, it's about minimizing permanent creases without making your face expressionless.

If you managed to get away with bad habits in your teens and 20s, those days are over. Late nights, smoking, excessive alcohol, unhealthy food, lack of exercise—all of this will take a huge toll on your skin now. Yet it's not too late to make changes, both in your lifestyle and your skin.

The Pregnancy Years

Now, some of you will sail through your pregnancy looking gorgeous, having that "glow" that people can see from a mile away. Be thankful if that's you . . . it certainly wasn't me. I had a heck of a time feeling beautiful while I was pregnant, since I had a pretty rough go of things. First off, I got toxemia, which is a pretty serious situation, and I also gained 65 pounds! So here's my advice to keep you feeling good, as well as to get that glow if it's just not happening for you naturally.

I've found that when you're having a baby, hormonal changes cause your skin to get either really good or really bad. It's tough if you have breakouts, because there are products and ingredients you really can't use when you're pregnant and breast-feeding, such as benzoyl peroxide and vitamin A products. You can try going natural with tea-tree oil, which is a mild antibacterial, and other ingredients are just fine. These include alpha hydroxy acids and fruit enzymes so that you can keep up with your exfoliation, as well as hyaluronic acid for hydrating.

As many as 70 percent of women get some melasma, which, as I've already mentioned, is also called pregnancy masking. These patches of pigmentation on your face (and other body parts) are caused by your hormones temporarily increasing melanin production. Make sure you exfoliate and wear a good sunscreen. In fact, I typically tell anyone who's pregnant to avoid sun exposure. (When I got pregnant, I instinctively didn't want anything to do with the sun.) Once you're done with your pregnancy and breast-feeding, you can really address the melasma issue with good results. Treatment options include the Pearl laser, Cosmelan, and peels.

Finally, while there isn't specific research that states these ingredients are harmful to use while pregnant, I suggest that the following be avoided: vitamin A (retinoids), salicylic acid, fragrance, hydrocortisone, and benzoyl peroxide.

40s

Cell turnover has slowed down quite a bit now, and you may even have cell damage. As for sun damage, that will really start to manifest now. I'm just heading into this age group, for instance, and I can see that all of the baking I did when I was younger has left patches of pigmentation lurking there on my skin, ready to come out. I found this out when I went under the Wood's lamp, a device that shows sun damage under the surface.

I'll have women of this age come in to the clinic and say, "I went to Hawaii, and these dark spots just appeared." Well, it wasn't their latest vacation that caused the spots. The sun may make them appear darker, but those spots formed when they were baking with tinfoil and iodine in their teens. This is where we have to use Retin-A to speed up cell turnover to get rid of that damage deep in the layers of the skin. Peptides are critical now, too.

Rosacea doesn't have an age limit—it's more of a hereditary issue—but typically it gets worse now as skin becomes thinner. You might see vascular problems for the same reason.

In your late 40s, you can start having hormonal issues as you approach perimenopause. Many women get breakouts again; if this does indeed happen to you, you'll be back to using acne medication, but just on the relevant areas.

While lines might have started forming in your 20s and 30s, now is when you start to see laxity. Titan is your treatment of choice for that because it's fantastic for tightening everything up. But the whole range of treatment options—lights, lasers, Botox, injectable fillers—is now going to benefit you more than anyone.

I'm a big believer in supplementing with vitamins, minerals, and omega-3 fatty acids now. And exercise and a good diet are absolutely the fountains of youth at this age.

50s

Menopause is the defining occurrence in this decade. Oh my goodness, anything can happen now: Estrogen and progesterone levels drop like a stone, which results in your making less and less collagen and elastin. Your skin thins and becomes drier. The decline in female hormones leaves testosterone more dominant, and you might have a recurrence of acne, along with the growth of facial hair. Subcutaneous fat degenerates and your muscles become more lax, causing sagging.

The joke of course is that nature causes our eyesight to get weaker as all of this stuff happens to our face so that we can remain blissfully ignorant! I'd recommend investing in one of those large, lighted, magnifying mirrors so you can see what's going on . . . and you'll spot those stray chin hairs that you need to take care of. As a bonus, those mirrors are great for applying makeup or shaping your eyebrows when you need reading glasses to see the small stuff.

The common denominator at this age is dryness. Topically, you can get rid of it through exfoliation and hydration. But now, the internal component is all the more important. This is when you need to make sure that you're supplementing to get the nutrients you need, especially the omegas. And I recommend taking internal hyaluronic acid and glucosamine, too. Adult acne can be treated with lights and topicals, but if there was ever a time to listen to my instruction to only use acne products on the affected sites, this is it.

You are a great candidate for the Pearl laser to resurface your skin and remove pigmentation and textural problems. Titan is also perfect for you to deal with the laxity. And you can see incredible results with injectable fillers like Juvéderm, Radiesse, and Cosmoplast, which will plump out those areas that have become hollow and gaunt looking. Combine them with artfully placed Botox, and you can take ten years off of your face without looking like you've done anything at all.

This is not the time to slack off on your physical activity—now more than ever, you need the blood and oxygen flow to your skin that vigorous exercise provides. By now the kids might be out of the house, so you should have the time to devote to exercising for your health.

60s and Beyond

The same regimens you develop in your 50s will take you through the following decades. But your skin will become increasingly thinner and drier, so you'll need to reevaluate from time to time to make sure that you're getting the hydration you need.

Pigmentation can become more apparent now, and sunscreen remains a must. Also, keep an eye on any moles that might be changing in shape, size, or color; these will need to be checked by a dermatologist because nonmelanoma cancers are most common in this age group.

Pay attention to your hair, teeth, and nails because they can betray your age, even when you have more youthful-looking skin. And don't get stuck in a time warp! Many women cling stubbornly to the look they had when they felt "in their prime," but it only serves to date them. Professional estheticians and hairstylists are your friends now and will keep you looking current.

You might be looking at retiring from work, so you'd have the time to devote to exercising and pursuing your passions, as well as rewarding yourself with pampering: a facial, massage, soak in the tub, or weekend trip to a spa with your friends.

Skin-telligence:

HUMIDIFIER HELP. If you live in an arid climate or have eczema or very dry skin, I highly recommend sleeping with a humidifier in the bedroom. It will significantly increase the moisture content of the air, which will add moisture to your skin and help relieve dryness. Additionally, if you have trouble sleeping, add a few drops of therapeutic essential oils to the water. Try chamomile, mandarin, or frankincense—all of which possess properties to promote restful sleep.

Most important, I want to stress that it's never too late to start taking care of your skin, nor are you ever too old to gain benefits from the wonderful products and treatments available today. The whole gamut of treatments is still available to you. Remember Fay McCallister from our makeover section? She's 71. Just look at the transformation in her!

◇◇◇

I do want to make it clear here that not everyone is going to want to do all of the treatments I mentioned in this chapter. Many people just want to take care of their skin so it remains healthy, but they opt not to have treatments and injections. That is a personal and an absolutely legitimate choice. I always honor whatever decision my clients make and never try to talk them into having something they don't want. After all, there is something to be said for aging gracefully, and legendary actress Lauren Bacall is the spokesperson for that philosophy. "I think your whole life shows in your face and you should be proud of that."

There's a Time and a Place

I want to address how to tweak your regimen according to where you live and the time of year. Some things are pretty obvious: If you live in an area with a very humid climate such as Florida, you don't need too much in the way of moisturization or heavy creams. But if you live somewhere like Arizona, the desert air sucks your skin dry and you desperately need all the hydration you can get. The same applies to terrains: the coastal Northwest has a lot more moisture in the air than a high mountain location like Colorado, which is incredibly dry, does.

In between all of those extremes, most of us live in climates that change seasonally, and there is a right time and a wrong time to get your treatments:

— *Winter.* I like to do my skin "work" in the winter months. I'm talking about peels and anything invasive that can strip away my protective layer or that might cause pigment changes. That would be IPL, peels, the Pearl laser, and so forth. There are two reasons for this. One is that it's important to avoid strong sun exposure after these treatments. The other is that I get to work on turning over any cell damage I might have done the previous summer.

I also recommend using glycolic acids and retinols in the winter, and hydrating really well. Making sure to get those omegas in your diet is important to boost your skin hydration. Also, because the weather is cold outside and warm inside, skin can get confused and parched.

— *Summer*. Summer is more about protective things like vitamin C serums that defend you against free-radical damage. Your summer regimen should be to hydrate with light moisturizers, exfoliate, and use sunscreen and self-tanners.

Piling on sunscreen can tend to clog pores, so it's also key to step up your facial regimen. If you don't normally get facials, it's not a bad idea to do a few during the summer months, so that debris doesn't clog and stretch pores or cause breakouts. It's okay to have light treatments and the Titan laser if you want, as they have no side effects. And drink lots of water to stay hydrated from the inside.

While we're on the subject of when to do things, I have one last important tip for you: *Never have a new procedure or treatment, or begin using a new product, right before some big occasion. You don't know how you're skin is going to react to it.* A red, irritated face or even an outbreak of hives is not the look you're going for at your prom, wedding, or job interview.

I had a celebrity client call me one morning, freaking out. She'd used a different eye cream (not mine!) the night before, and when she woke up, her eyes were swollen, puffy, red, irritated, and itchy. She had a photo shoot that day, so she frantically asked, "What do I do?!" To be honest, there's very little you can do with such a reaction. I told her to take an antihistamine to reduce the swelling, and to place cotton balls soaked in ice water on the eyes.

Here's my advice: Test a new product three to four weeks before something important. That way, there's time for your skin to calm down.

I've got some more tips for you, in the form of questions my team and I hear all the time in our clinic. Just turn the page to be enlightened!

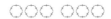

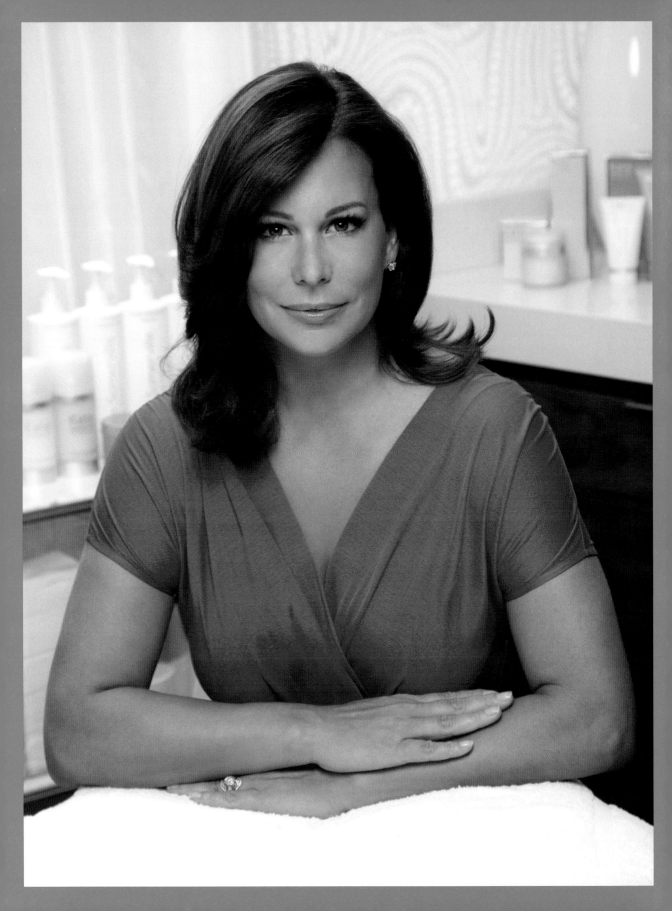

CHAPTER 11

Quiz Kate!
Questions Answered

My clinic is made up of some of the most dedicated and talented estheticians and nurses you'll find anywhere: they really are the "Skin Health Experts." On any given day, each one of them can see seven to ten clients. That's about 80 women a day. Seven days a week. Four weeks a month. And let me tell you, we women can talk— and we women have questions about our skin. Lots of them!

So I asked my team to make me a list of the common questions they get all of the time and to include some of the more unusual ones. I also added my own. After all, when I'm not at my clinic, I'm frequently doing personal appearances with our retailers, and sometimes I'll consult with 45 different women in one day, checking out their skin . . . and boy, talk about questions!

I've gathered all of the good ones my team and I have heard and compiled them in this chapter. I know that we've already discussed so many aspects of skin health in this book, but I wanted to make sure to answer any questions you may have that haven't come up so far. Hopefully, something you've always wondered about will be addressed in the next eight pages. Here we go!

Q: Does Preparation H® work to reduce puffiness, dark circles, and tired eyes?

A: Preparation H contains an ingredient—phenylephrine—that constricts blood vessels and causes tissue to temporarily contract and tighten. This squeezes the fluid out of skin tissue and therefore can reduce puffiness. The contraction of the vessels can also make dark circles less apparent. However, this product is not formulated for the delicate eye area and can cause irritation, so use with caution.

Q: Why do I have so many blackheads on my nose, and how can I get rid of them?

A: Ugh! Blackheads are a very common problem, especially on the nose: this center of the T-zone has a very high concentration of oil glands. These glands get congested easily, filling with blackheads and stretching pores.

To keep blackheads from forming on the nose, start by getting a facial, and ask your facialist to concentrate on unplugging those clogged pores. Once they're clean, work to keep them that way. Exfoliate once or twice a week to prevent dead skin cells from clogging pores and trapping oil. (The Clarisonic brush my clinicians use can work wonders on blackheads, too.) Finally, doing a light at-home peel once a week can also help kill bacteria inside pores and dissolve excess oil. This will prevent those pesky blackheads from forming. An over-the-counter treatment product that contains glycolic or lactic acid is a good choice—my favorites are the Kate Somerville Micro Lactic Polisher and the Micro Glycolic Polisher.

Q: There are these tiny hard, white bumps on my face—they aren't like regular whiteheads, are stubborn, and won't go away. What are they, and how can I get rid of them?

A: Most likely, those little bumps are milia, which occur when oil and debris become trapped beneath the surface of the skin. The gunk isn't actually in the pores, so it doesn't have an escape route.

Milia are particularly common around the eyes, usually caused by too-rich creams. It's better to use a light eye cream with effective ingredients rather than a really thick, rich cream that may moisturize but will also congest. Also, look to see if your eye-makeup remover has mineral oil in it, since that's a big culprit as well.

If you try to get to your milia yourself, you could damage the tissue. Instead, please go to your dermatologist or esthetician to have them extracted.

Q: If my foundation has sun protection, do I still need to wear sunscreen underneath?

A: If your makeup has an SPF of 15 or higher, that should be enough coverage for your average day, as long as you evenly apply it all over your skin. However, keep in mind that you're probably not applying this foundation on your neck, chest, and hands, so make sure to apply sunscreen to those areas to ensure the best protection.

Q: The skin on my eyelids frequently gets itchy, dry—even flaky—and swollen. How should I treat this, and how can I prevent it?

A: I suffer from this problem myself, and it can be hard to figure out. Eyelid skin is much thinner than other areas, has very little protective fat, and is more vascular; this makes the tissue more sensitive and prone to allergies and irritants. I recommend taking an antihistamine to reduce the redness, irritation, and swelling. Also, it's important to keep the area hydrated with a basic moisturizer that won't aggravate the delicate tissue. I like to use Traumeel, a homeopathic ointment, around my own eyes when they're irritated.

If your irritation is very bad, I recommend going to the ophthalmologist or dermatologist for a topical steroid prescription. If the problem occurs often, it's worth getting to the bottom of what's causing it. You may want to have an allergy patch test done to determine specific allergies. Common culprits can include contact-lens solutions, cosmetics, skin-care products, metals, glues, and hair colorants.

Q: I always seem to break out in the same exact spot. Why does that happen, and what can I do to prevent it?

A: Some experts believe that recurring breakouts on specific areas of the face can reflect the health of particular organs, and I believe that this is a possibility. Certainly, it's not uncommon for breakouts around the chin and jawline to reflect a hormonal imbalance and problems with the female reproductive organs. It's never a bad idea to look into the health and welfare of your body and organs if you consistently break out in certain spots.

If your breakouts are mild, I recommend prevention by spot treating the area every other night with a salicylic-acid lotion or gel, and using a clay mask a few times a week.

Q: I've started exercising more and have been getting little bumps and irritations on my forehead. In general, my skin looks healthier, but these breakouts are really bothering me. What's happening?

A: It's very important to always splash water on your face before leaving the gym or the yoga studio. This will help prevent dirt, oil, and sweat from settling into your pores and creating buildup, breakouts, and irritation. Also, rigorous exercise encourages detoxification, so you may be noticing the release of toxins through your skin, which is normal—and good for you.

Q: I never had large pores, but as I get older, they seem to be getting more noticeable. Why is that, and what can I do?

A: Pore size is more or less genetic, and unless you do a series of pretty intense laser treatments and peels, it's not realistic to get rid of sizable ones. However, even if you didn't inherit large pores, they can get bigger as you age due to loss of elasticity. It's most important to clear them and tighten your skin to keep your complexion looking as smooth as possible. Use products with gentle acids (such as lactic or glycolic) a few times a week. Retin-A is also great for keeping pores clear and stimulating collagen and elastin to tighten pores over time.

Q: I've heard so many horror stories about lasers. How do I know if where I'm going to get treatment is safe?

A: Every state has different laws regarding lasers, so do your research. You can often go to the Better Business Bureau Website to investigate the place you want to go for treatment and learn about its customer satisfaction and ethics. And always have a consultation first. Speak to the nurse or the doctor—ask questions, and don't be afraid to ask if they've had problems in the past; how long they've been in business; and what you should realistically expect regarding results. While lasers are generally safe and effective, it's important to find a technician who's highly trained, skilled, and confident. *Find someone you can trust.* I cannot express the importance of this enough.

Q: There are so many types of exfoliants—enzymes, acids, microdermabrasions. Do I need to do them all?

A: My team and I get this question a lot. Exfoliants are like veggies in that there are so many. Do you need to eat them all to be healthy? No, but you should eat a variety. I feel that variety is also the key to exfoliants: enzymes are great because they gently dissolve the dead cells, microbeads help slough away those cells, and AHAs and BHAs work on different levels to do the same thing. Alternating all of these exfoliants prevents your body from getting used to one so that they continue to work efficiently. So my answer is that it's good to use a few different methods, as long as they're gentle as well as effective. Switch it up!

Q: I have some white spots and patches on my skin. What are they?

A: White patches are complicated and can be caused by a variety of reasons. Sometimes loss of pigment is a postinflammatory response—there may have been severe or recurring irritation to the skin, and this is the result. It's really stubborn, and those of us in the skin-care field are still looking for ways to stimulate pigment production where it's been lost.

Then there is a different condition called vitiligo, which is genetic. It usually appears in symmetrical patches around the eyes and on the legs and elbows, and it's often found on the hands. Dermatologists are experimenting with different creams, but a truly effective solution has yet to be developed.

Q: Is it really a big deal to go to bed without washing off my makeup? Sometimes I get home and am just too tired.

A: If it's a once-in-a-blue-moon occurrence, then that's okay. But if this is a habit, your complexion will appear dull and less healthy. Buildup will develop and can clog pores, causing your skin to look lifeless. It's important to wash before bed. If you do that—and if your skin is really balanced and healthy—it's not always essential to wash your face with cleanser in the morning. Instead, just go ahead and splash with cold water and then moisturize.

Q: As I get older, my skin is getting more sensitive. Is this normal?

A: Yes. As we age, our skin cells tend to turn over less frequently. So if we have an irritation or a breakout, it tends to heal more slowly. Our skin cells also tend to thin out, which can leave skin more sensitive.

As you get older, it's important to reevaluate your products and treatment regimen. You may realize that certain products and ingredients that you could use when you were younger are now too strong for your changing skin.

Q: Are preservatives like parabens harmful to us and our bodies?

A: Most skin-care products contain preservatives, which help prevent the growth of bacteria and fungi that would otherwise contaminate and spoil them. Parabens are some of the most common classes of preservatives and include methylparaben, propylparaben, and butylparaben. A 2002 study found parabens in breast tissue, which ignited fear that they could cause breast cancer; however, the study did not actually show that connection. It's not even known whether the topical application of parabens is what leads to their accumulation in our bodies.

Parabens can cause reactions in people with active eczema, or in those allergic to these compounds. The rest of us can be guided by the conclusion published in 2006 by the FDA that cosmetics containing parabens are safe. Yet because there has been so much about this in the media, we're currently taking parabens out of the Kate Somerville product collection to assuage concerns that some individuals still have.

Q: I have little bumps that don't itch up and down the backs of my arms. I've had them since I was little, and I can't seem to get my skin smooth, no matter what I do.

A: Exfoliation and hydration is the answer. My team and I have had a lot of clients enjoy tremendous success in getting rid of these annoying bumps simply by using my ExfoliKate enzyme scrub combined with my Goat Milk Body Lotion. The exfoliant eats away the dead skin cells, and the goat milk softens the skin and reduces the bumps, treating them with the gentle, naturally occurring lactose enzyme in the lotion.

Q: Does sleeping on your side cause wrinkles?

A: Yes, it does. In fact, there are some dermatologists and skin-care specialists who can tell which side you sleep on because of how your wrinkles have formed. Not only do you get facial wrinkles, but if you have a big bust, you'll also get creases on your chest. To help with that, you can try sleeping with a small pillow between your breasts. But the only real answer is to sleep on your back.

Q: Is men's skin different from women's?

A: No: Skin is skin. Sometimes it might seem that they're different because men don't typically apply all of the ingredients that women do (although that is changing somewhat). Of course they do shave, so they can have problems such as razor burn or ingrown hairs. But the skin structure is exactly the same.

Q: When I'm applying serums and moisturizers, should I just glide them on top of my skin or rub them in?

A: You should gently massage them in. If the product is something with a treatment in it, you want to move it into the skin so that it can really absorb. The thicker the cream or lotion, the more you need to smooth it in because the ingredient is suspended in oils and will just sit on the surface of your skin if you don't dissolve the oil. Just be sure not to tug and pull your skin.

Q: I'm very red around the creases of my nostrils. What is this, and how can I treat it?

A: These are broken capillaries and fairly easy to treat with a laser. The heat will cauterize the capillary, shrinking it down, and it will feel like a very warm rubber-band snap. Depending on the size, you may need several treatments, and they can come back over time. However, please be sure to find a doctor or medical spa that has performed this treatment many times, as selecting an expert with experience is crucial in this case.

Q: What causes cold sores, and what can I do about them?

A: Cold sores on your face are usually herpes simplex virus type 1. Once you've contracted the virus, it can be triggered by sun exposure, stress, trauma, or food sensitivities (lactose and glucose are common ones). Some clinical treatments like lasers and topicals such as retinol can also cause an outbreak. Taking supplements of l-lysine, an amino acid, seems to retard the frequency of outbreaks. Once you feel the tingling of a sore coming on, immediately apply one of the topical depressant medications available in drugstores. Applying aloe-vera gel can help keep the sore lubricated and may even help speed recovery. Do *not* pick the sore—and since herpes is extremely infectious, don't kiss anyone until it's gone!

Q: What causes dark circles under eyes? Is there something preventive I can be doing to keep them at bay?

A: Lifestyle factors such as smoking, drinking alcohol, not getting enough sleep, and eating poorly can contribute. The natural aging process is also a common reason: loss of collagen and fat leaves skin thinner, making blood vessels more apparent. Because blood is blue in our bodies, this area appears bluish. Sometimes pigmentation is caused by the sun; certain medications may be the culprit; or the circles are simply inherited.

For thinning skin, I recommend eye creams with peptides to boost collagen. Lasers can help, and my favorite is Laser Genesis for this. If pigmentation is the problem, lightening creams may work, but you have to be careful around the sensitive eye area; IPL treatment may also help reduce pigment. Oxygen facials are good for stimulating circulation, which may improve the condition of those whose circles are caused by stagnated blood flow, frequently the result of lack of sleep, stress, or sinus congestion. Most important, always look at what is safest for you, because the tissue in this area is very delicate.

Now that my team and I have given you the benefit of our knowledge and experience, I'm going to hand you over to the Hollywood Glam Squad for the finishing touches!

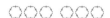

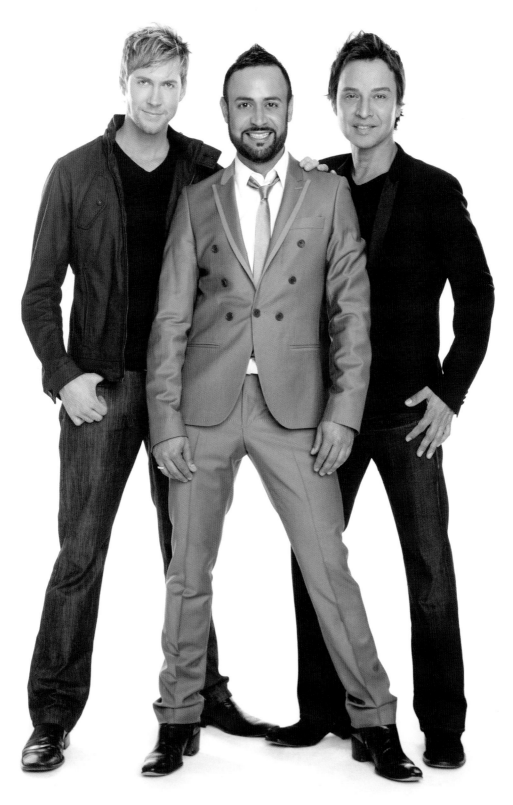

My Hollywood Glam Squad—Spencer Barnes: makeup;
Nick Verreos: fashion; and Darrell Redleaf: hair.

CHAPTER 12

My Hollywood Glam Squad

Getting celebrities ready for a special event where they'll be photographed is a lot of work. Yes, they always look amazing in photos. But guess what? They get help.

Sure, a lot of them are gorgeous to start, yet there's always an incredible amount of effort and collaboration behind celebrity style and "the look" that somehow seems to set them apart. The truth is, behind every on-screen talent, there is offscreen talent. I'm part of that behind-the-scenes team!

I'm ground zero: I work on the skin and try to perfect it, and then off my client goes to her hair, makeup, and fashion stylists. These talented artists help glamorize movie stars by dressing them, tressing them, painting them up, and teaching them how to do all of this for themselves.

I'm lucky to work with some of the most talented people in the beauty business, so I decided to collaborate with a few of these wonderful individuals to do a few head-to-toe makeovers on Lori, Shayne, and Fay, three of our volunteers from Part III. (Don't you skip ahead and sneak a peek!)

These three ladies are typical of so many of the clients in this book who shared with me how much of an impact changing their skin had made on them, both inside and out. The external transformation was feeding a positive internal metamorphosis that seemed to brighten every corner of each of their lives, and they were feeling much better about themselves all around. I wanted to go a step further and give them the tools to see their *total* potential.

First I called Spencer Barnes, a close friend and an incredible makeup artist, to see if he'd do the makeup. Then I called Darrell Redleaf, hands down one of the most genius hair guys in Hollywood, to see if he'd take care of the tresses. And last—but never least—I called Nick Verreos, who possesses the most flawless sense of fashion I've ever seen, to see if he'd handle the clothes and accessories for the resulting photo shoot. Happily, they all said yes.

Sometimes people don't even know that their hairstyle is aging them or that the color of their clothes is washing them out. I can work on their skin, but if they choose to wear something that doesn't complement them, their skin can look less healthy and vibrant (and honestly, older). Maybe they don't know how to accent their eyes or bring attention to their best features. Or maybe they'd just like a little change or an update, but they're just not sure how to do it—or at least how to do it well. Enter the Hollywood Glam Squad! These experts spent a day with Fay, Lori, and Shayne, showing them how to put together a polished look that was still true to who they were. I honestly love these women, and I even love their "before" pictures, but for me, it was so much fun to see what the Glam Squad created for them. All of them now have "that look" that sets them apart. Wow! If I've learned anything from this experience, it's that transforming someone's outside can truly transform the person on the inside, too. I hope you can find that for yourself as well.

In the following pages, you'll meet the special guys in the Glam Squad; learn their valuable insider tips; and see what amazing things they've done with Fay, Lori, and

Shayne. It is with great pride that I turn the rest of the chapter over to these amazing men. (Each one of them has his own section, which is written in his own voice.) I now leave you in their capable hands, and I'll meet back up with you in the Afterword.

SPENCER BARNES: MAKEUP ARTIST

Even though I've crafted looks for celebrities for red-carpet appearances, music videos, editorials, press junkets, ad campaigns, fashion runways, television, and film, I always love the opportunity to work with "everyday" women.

Early in my makeup career, I traveled around the western U.S. as a national makeup artist for Lancôme, hosting cosmetic-counter events. I worked one-on-one with thousands of women and discovered just how vulnerable many of them feel when barefaced. I believe that all people have inherent beauty, and one of my loves in life is to show them this beauty. When I transform a woman and give her fuller lips or longer lashes, it's great, but what's truly remarkable is what happens to her inner confidence. How she feels about herself comes through in every aspect of her life.

Through my gift of makeup, I can help you see yourself in a new way and portray this to others. Makeup is an extension of the self: with it, you can be a smoldering temptress one day and a soft coquette the next. It's these transformations and looks that give me great satisfaction as a makeup artist. So now I'd like to share some tips with you that you can easily do for yourself.

BROW WOW!

Although beauty begins with clear and healthy skin, nothing can transform and improve a face more than well-shaped eyebrows. For starters, focus less on how thick or thin your brows are and more on improving their overall shape and structure, as that's more important and achievable by everyone:

— Brush brows in the direction of hair growth, or slightly down, and assess them. Study the natural shape and proportion of your brows, along with the color and length of the hairs.

— Consider the shape. The brow should begin above the inner corner of your eye, the arch should be about three-quarters of the way across, and the brow should extend just beyond the outside corner of your eye.

— After you've brushed your brows, you may want to gently trim if there are any long or unruly hairs that extend beyond the natural shape. Use fingernail scissors and caution. Tweeze any fine hairs between the brow and the lid and any that are outside of the natural shape.

— Now it's time to shade. For thinner brows, find a powder or brow pencil one to two shades lighter than your natural hair color. This way, you'll add depth to the brow without drawing attention to the presence of product. If in doubt about which color is best for you, taupe is a good option for most hair colors. If your brows are too far apart, fill in a little here (also, be sure to fill in any gaps or holes). Tinted brow-grooming gels are a great way to add a little color and help unruly hairs stay in place. For women with hair tones in the red/auburn family, a red-based brow gel will really make the eyes, hair, and skin pop.

— If you chemically alter your hair color and it's significantly different from your natural brow shade, you may want to have them professionally colored to complement your hair (notice how we lightened Shayne's brows in her makeover).

CONCEAL TO REVEAL

This is such an important step. Concealer corrects imperfections and discoloration, brightens and balances, and can be used to manipulate your facial features. If you get it right, you can leave the house with just this product and a little mascara. Here's how to use it like an expert:

— Choose the correct shade. Many women make a mistake and end up looking like they've been skiing in the sun wearing goggles. If the area under your eyes is paler than the rest of your face, try using a shade that's just a bit darker to blend them together. If your undereye area is darker, you'll definitely want a shade that lightens or brightens. Take a flash photo if you're not sure.

— Prepare your skin by applying moisturizer. Then apply a "swoosh" (like the Nike logo) of concealer under your eyes. You can use a brush or your fourth or pinky finger to blend.

— I like to apply a brighter, lighter shade down the bridge of the nose, between the brows, and at the top of the cheekbones because it adds dimension to the face. Work this into the skin for a seamless blend.

— For spots or blemishes, dab a shade that matches your tone (or one darker) onto the spot. It's best to use a brush for this.

— Always set concealer with translucent powder.

— Generally, if you want to brighten a sallow complexion or have too much yellow in your skin, balance with a concealer and foundation that has a subtle lavender tone. If you have too much redness, look for a product with more beige or yellow.

FOUNDATION FACTS

You may not need foundation. But if you require some coverage, it can help you fake a flawless complexion while you're still working on your skin. I know that Kate loves mineral foundation, but I tend to like liquid. One isn't necessarily better than the other; go with the one that suits you best. Here's the best way to apply it:

— For lighter skin tones, match the foundation to the side of your cheek or jawline. Don't match to the cheek where the skin tends to be pinker. Look in natural light and watch for the undertones.

— Darker skin types tend to be darker around the perimeter of the face and brighter in the center. You want to match foundation to your forehead or nose.

— You don't always need to put foundation over your entire face. Using a foundation brush, apply a small amount that you've warmed on the back of your hand so that it will go on smoothly. Blend in with your fingers, and let your natural undertones show through.

— Use a large, soft, round brush to dust on a translucent powder to set liquid and cream makeup, particularly in hot and humid climates.

LET THERE BE LIGHT

Illuminating your face with light and delicate shading can enhance every feature and create a special luminosity:

— Pick a neutral highlight color and apply under the eyebrow and on the brow bone. You can do this with a pale cream or powder concealer.

— Highlighting just under and above the arch of the brow with a powder that is one or two shades lighter than the natural skin tone will look natural, but make your eyes pop.

— Tired eyes? Add a bit of shimmer or pearl color in the center of the lid, above the lash line, or in the corner.

— Feel free to use bronzer, which can add dimension and enhance bone structure, but easy does it! Think about where the sun would hit your face naturally: the bridge of your nose, your hairline, a little on your neck. And be sure to blend down into your chest to avoid a color contrast with your face and neck.

ESSENTIALS FOR EYES

The eyes are the most expressive part of the face. So first think, what message do you want to send? Once you've decided that, you can get to work:

— If you plan on using a lot of shadows, prep the lid with an eye-shadow base. This way, the shadow won't crease and will last.

— In general, earth tones— browns, peaches, beiges, creams, chocolates, bronzes— are going to look the most natural. For drama without committing to color, silver, gray, charcoal, pewter, and taupe all work well.

— Color can be a lot of fun and doesn't have to read "heavy." For example, if your eyes are brown, a sweep of lavender liner or shadow can be a simple way to really make a statement. Just make sure to smudge at the lash line and transition colors by blending.

— When using liner on the top lid, always work it into the lash line, making sure not to leave a gap. On the bottom, a perfect line can look hard—gently soften with a cotton swab or try stippling (that is, using small dots or strokes) it into the lower lash line. And for a smoky look, use a small "smudger" brush and blend the creamy pencil into the lashes. Add a little powder of the same color to take it a step further and to set the liner.

— Lash but not least: Curl your lashes before you put on mascara. It will instantly open up your eyes. Then an even sweep of lash primer or even a dusting of powder can help boost lash volume. Work the mascara in, starting at the base of the lashes, moving the wand back and forth as you extend toward the tips. This helps separate the lashes and deposits color at the base. If you want more volume, add a second or third coat, but make sure to have a lash comb handy to separate lashes and prevent clumping.

— Remember balance. If you're going for a dark or smoldering eye, for instance, opt for a softer lip to allow the eyes to take the lead. If you're using white eye shadow, a deeper lip color is a good idea.

TIPS FOR LIPS

Next to eyes, your lips are the second most expressive feature on your face. So pay attention to the preparation, because like it or not, lips are moving and are automatically going to draw attention:

— After you've brushed your teeth and had your kiss good night, apply a hydrating balm or lip treatment to prepare the area. Five years of no lip care will definitely lead to that feathery lip line. (Just ask Kate!)

— Gone are the days of lining your lips with a highly pigmented liner. Instead, try this: grab a nude lip liner with a hint of pearl or light, as this will enhance the natural shape of your lip. And then apply your gloss or lipstick of choice on top.

—If you aren't a strong-lip-color person, there are so many great balms that give just a hint of tint and can really make a face look younger, healthy, and fresh.

— When in doubt, a soft, fleshy pink or warm coral looks good on almost everyone.

— If you finish your lip color with a brush of sheer powder, you'll get more staying power.

MAGIC TRICKS

Here are a few little tricks I use to make a celebrity look like a celebrity. They are simple and easy, and you can do them, too!

— I love adding lashes, which you can find in beauty-supply shops or drugstores. You don't necessarily have to use a full strip; individual flares or single lashes work just fine. I'll put them in the center of the eye for a doe-eyed look, or toward outer edges for a sexier, elongated eye. Don't be afraid to experiment with lashes, as they can look very natural but still add drama.

— Sometimes I'll use a bronzy brown or burgundy mascara on the bottom lashes to add color but keep the eyes soft. This makes eye color pop.

— Line the underside of the eye—under the top lashes, or above the bottom ones—with liner. Try black and charcoal for drama, or gold and silver for an extra dimension.

— Don't be afraid to try a little contouring. If you're going to have your picture taken, it's really important because features tend to lose strength in photos. To do this naturally, you can use two different foundations: slightly lighter in the center, and darker around the perimeter. Blush and bronzer work to add dimension, too.

— Cheeks are a major part of your face, so play them up! It's always safe to choose a pink, coral, or bronze tone. If you aren't applying blush, you should be. It will make your eyes and smile dazzle.

— Adding a little bronzer will instantly wake up the face. But please, back away from the "tanorexia" look: You don't want it to look like you've got a tanning machine parked out back!

— Microglitter is great for live occasions but not for photography. I'll use it on the eyes or lips. It's great in low light settings and can be so visually compelling.

DARRELL REDLEAF: HAIRSTYLIST

I've been doing hair ever since I can remember. I can hardly believe it myself, but I've been a hairstylist in the entertainment industry for almost 25 years! As you can imagine, I've seen three decades of trends, from '70s disco hair, '80s mullets and permed hair, and '90s natural straight hair to the current voluminous, wavy, sexy styles.

I have an extensive celebrity clientele, which I've garnered over the years. Because I'm truly interested in all things beauty, I also frequently serve as a beauty expert and correspondent in the media. I'm often asked, "How do the stars always look so put together?"

My answer is, "Believe me, you'd look good, too, if you had a brigade of people hired to do just that. Smoke and mirrors, baby!"

Everyone starts out the same in the morning. No one looks like a glamorous movie star when there's a 4 A.M. call time on the set, especially when they went partying and got home three hours ago! But it's my job to create incredible looks every day. They can be simple or dramatic. But the truth is, healthy, gorgeous hair takes work and care just like with the skin.

THE FOUR C'S

When clients ask me, "What should I do with my hair?" My answer usually is, "What are you doing with your hair?"

Make a hair assessment. Every detail is contingent on every other detail. When considering your hair, particularly its styling and care, where are you coming from? Where are you now? And where are you going? My advice is based on my own hair system: **the four C's: clarify, condition, color,** and **cut.** Here's a detailed explanation of each:

1. CLARIFY

Literally and figuratively, **clarify** means "to make clear." Most of you probably overcondition, overprocess, overdry, overcolor, and overstress your hair. And when you're drying, curling, or flatironing your hair, understand that you're baking all of this into your hair shaft: products, medications you've taken, and impurities and pollutants from the environment.

Imagine laying coat after coat of wax on your kitchen floor or on the surface of your car. Hair is the same, except it's porous. Hairs lay on top of each other, and when they're exploded by bleaching, coloring, drying, ironing, or curling, their first layer—the cuticle layer—is fried. Everything that goes onto the hair gets absorbed by it, and these impurities eventually become baked in. A clarifier will remove the product buildup—the junk, the pollutants, the medications, and the waxes from overconditioning.

I recommend clarifying at least once a month. It's like a facial for the hair. There are many products and shampoos on the market that can do the job, but believe it or not, the simplest and easiest is an apple-cider-vinegar rinse.

2. CONDITION

Just like our skin craves to be moisturized, our hair needs to **condition** itself, or drink water, too. Hydration is key to beautiful hair, so not only should we drink plenty of water every day, we also need to find a product that will hydrate and protect our locks externally.

I don't recommend washing and conditioning your hair every day because that's too much stress on it. I'll give you the same advice that I generally give my clients: go into the two-day cycle. Wash and condition your hair every other day, and on the off days, just get under the shower stream and scrub your hair like you have a lather going. You'll remove product and the daily accumulation of debris in the hair, but you won't strip out the natural oils that your hair needs.

The only exception is if your hair is extremely oily. In that case, I suggest using a weekly deep conditioner. If you leave it on for several minutes, it will hydrate the hair and penetrate more deeply.

When looking for a conditioner, even the most expensive can create buildup. So it's recommended to switch back and forth between two lines. But if you're clarifying your hair once a month or so, this should keep your hair healthy and you should be fine.

3. COLOR

Hair **color** is a very personal and specific choice. But that choice can have a dramatic effect on how your skin looks—it can make your complexion look great, or it can actually make it appear unhealthy. So when selecting a hair color, you need to select something that truly complements your skin, rather than going after the latest fashion. My vision of beautiful hair color comes from nature, and everyone starts off with a natural hair color. In order to enhance that color, it's generally best to consult with a reputable hair colorist before attempting to change it, highlight it, or cover up the gray. A good colorist will always consider your skin tone when helping you make a selection, and do find someone you like and trust.

I've repaired so many botched hair-color jobs, either from inexperienced stylists or from clients testing the waters at home on their own. My personal recommendation is to never change your base color, unless you have a lot of gray and need to bring it back to your original color. In that case, go for it. Otherwise, you'll most likely turn your base color into something that doesn't work with or balance the natural tones in your skin. And the point of hair color is to bring out and complement your natural features and skin tone.

I see so many women who want to be blonde or red, but they really should be choosing a color that matches their complexion. Blonde, auburn, or red hair next to a ruddy, pinkish complexion can actually make it look worse. A better option is a sandier color or ashy blonde, as this will neutralize the pink tones in the skin.

In my experience, the majority of people have yellow to green undertones in their skin color and medium to dark hair. If you have dark hair and eyes and want to go lighter, or even blonde, a yellow-toned blonde is not advisable. This will only make your skin tone look more sallow or custard colored, which is certainly not very flattering, and it will actually make you look older, too. But lightening and brightening *is* possible. For highlights, you can safely jump up two to three hair shades. Any more will look streaky and unnatural. The key is to always avoid brassiness or orange. If you're dark haired and want a lift, I recommend choosing a golden brown or a midtoned blonde, depending on the yellow undertones of your skin. Lighter hair shades can pull off a platinum blonde, but most others really need to steer clear. This color will emphasize imperfections in the skin.

4. CUT

As we all know, finding the correct **cut** is essential for the overall look we're trying to achieve—in combination with our color, this is what gives character to our hair. For most women today, hairstyling is about a wash-and-wear haircut. So, more than ever, the cut is crucial. I personally like to cut hair dry. That way, I can see how the haircut is coming out.

I do tell my clients to bring pictures of styles they like so that we can discuss the feasibility of that look on them. It really is so helpful, since their idea of golden highlights and fringe bangs may be entirely different from my vision.

Getting back to the cut, there are a few general concepts that tend to make sense. For example, a girl in her teens to 20s can have longer hair. From 30 on up, however, I look for styles and cuts that are a bit shorter, lighter, and freer. These rules aren't hard-and-fast, but if you're noticing the pull of gravity, a shorter style can add a visual lift to the face.

Face shape should always be considered as well, and a great stylist will know this naturally. A haircut can completely balance a face or distort it. If you have a larger forehead, bangs—be they short and choppy or long and sweeping—can set off your eyes and make your forehead appear more proportional. If you have a longer face shape, a shorter cut with full layers will help add width to the face. This is definitely something that can be worked out with your stylist. Talking these things out will help you get the result you want: one that highlights your personal style, adds to your confidence, and complements your skin.

NICK VERREOS: FASHION STYLIST

I've been involved with fashion all my life. As early as I can remember, I was always sketching women in stylish fashions. As a young child, my love of fashion was limited to the chic stewardesses (I know, we call them flight attendants now, but back in my "day," they were fabulous stewardesses) I saw so often. My father was a foreign-service attaché, so we traveled a lot. I was fascinated by these stewardesses and loved drawing them. I also always loved drawing my mom when she got ready for her black-tie diplomatic parties when we lived in Caracas, Venezuela.

I realize now that there are three things that made these women (the stewardesses and my mom) stand out. So here are my ABCs to being stylish and fabulous at any age:

A IS FOR ACCESSORIZE

The right accessories can make a world of difference in your overall style, especially when it comes to adding personality to your look. A bold necklace, an eye-catching bag, or a red python shoe—*faux,* of course—can change that "same old, same old" black shift dress from blah to fab in 1.2 seconds. (Okay, maybe three minutes is more likely.) If you wore that simple dress to the office under a jacket, all you'd have to do is remove the jacket, add a necklace with some heels and a clutch, and *voilà.* It will look like a whole new dress, and you'll look like a whole new you! Trust me on this one, ladies. A fantastic statement-making necklace can transform an outfit in a snap. It's also great for bringing the eye back to your beautiful face—and it's a way to start a conversation!

Think of accessories as investment pieces: Don't be afraid to spend some money on shoes, purses, and jewelry. You can wear accessories over and over again—with different garments—more easily than you can wear that same dress. For example, I bought a pair of *fierce* YSL men's boots, and yes, they were pricey, but I almost sleep in them! I wear them with every jean, jacket, and dress shirt I own.

B IS FOR BODY (AND, OF COURSE, FIT)

I cannot emphasize enough how important it is to know your body and what shapes work best for you. Are you a "balanced hourglass" (that 36-26-36 shape), "pear shaped" (little up top, wider at the bottom), "apple shaped" (wide all over), or just a stick (straight and narrow)? Here are some quick guidelines when it comes to different shapes:

— If you're wide at the bottom, keep the darks below the waist and the lighter, brighter colors up top. A flared black skirt paired with a colorful top and a fabulous necklace usually works with this body shape. If you're wider-hipped, stay away from the boot-cut or flared pant, as it will only emphasize your hips. Stick to a straight-leg pant, which will fall straight from your hips and thigh. And definitely do not do leggings or skinny jeans.

— For women with minimal busts, halter necklines are great; they emphasize the neck and shoulders and give an illusion of a fuller bust. Halter styles are also great for women with small shoulders in that they give the impression of being wider.

—More buxom women look great in wrap dresses and surplice tops (that go across the bust), as well as tops or dresses with an empire or underbust seam. Usually under the bust will be the smallest place on your body, so drawing attention to this area works to slim. A wrap dress takes the eye in a diagonal direction, creating a waist where there may be none, and it's one continuous look that does not break up the overall silhouette.

The second part of this tip is all about the fit. Designers and manufacturers of clothing make sizing according to a "balanced body," which is the standard in the industry. Think of the female dancers on *Dancing with the Stars* and their body shapes. Those dancers have a well-proportioned, size-4 shape: some bust, a defined waist, and hips the same size as their bust. Now grade their bodies up to that version of a 10, 12, or 14, and that is how clothes are built. But here's the deal: most women, or human beings for that matter, may not have a "balanced," well-proportioned body. That's why most of us should have a tailor or seamstress fit the clothes we buy to make them even better. For example, let's say that you're shopping for pants, and your hips fit a size 12 but your waist is an 8. Buy the 12, and get the waist tailored so that it fits you perfectly in the waist, too. This may take a little effort, but it's definitely worth the time and expense.

C IS FOR COLOR

Color is the punctuation mark in any woman's wardrobe. Everybody relies on the staples: black, gray, tan, and white. Why not add color to your wardrobe to inject some style? Keep the black suit or dress but add a colorful coat, top, or jacket to add some flair. I love it when I see a woman with a fantastic turquoise wool peacoat with a peek of a black dress underneath it. More often than not, I'll even go up to her and say, "I love your coat." Again, like jewelry and accessories, colored clothes demand conversation and can change an old stale outfit instantly. They're "item" pieces—go ahead and buy several of them.

Be bold with your color when you normally wouldn't be, especially if you're feeling—or looking—a little tired. Instead of that brown purse, go for an emerald green one. Instead of the navy wrap dress, go for a colorful printed one, à la Diane von Furstenberg, and watch how many compliments you'll get. The right color is an instant ego boost and will absolutely brighten up your face.

Now in terms of wearing color, there *are* some guidelines. Olive-toned women look best in the richer, primary colors and metallic hues, but don't always shine in drab, earth tones. Women with lighter complexions look great in pastels like violet, powder blue, and lemon yellow, but are overwhelmed by stronger colors such as fuchsia and chartreuse. Make sure to experiment and try on colors that you may not be used to wearing. You might be surprised by how good you actually look in it and how much it turned your look up a whole lot of notches!

Ultimately, a few of these easy fashion changes and additions can really help add spice to your entire presence. Glowing skin is always complemented by hues that bring out the natural color in your cheeks, or a neckline that sets off your complexion.

We had clothes generously lent to us by some designers and retailers for the photo shoot; we hope they inspire you. Having said that, know that you don't need to spend a lot of money to have a fashionable wardrobe that you can have fun with. If you play with a few of these ideas, you'll see just how simple and versatile your wardrobe and look can be.

Let the makeovers begin!

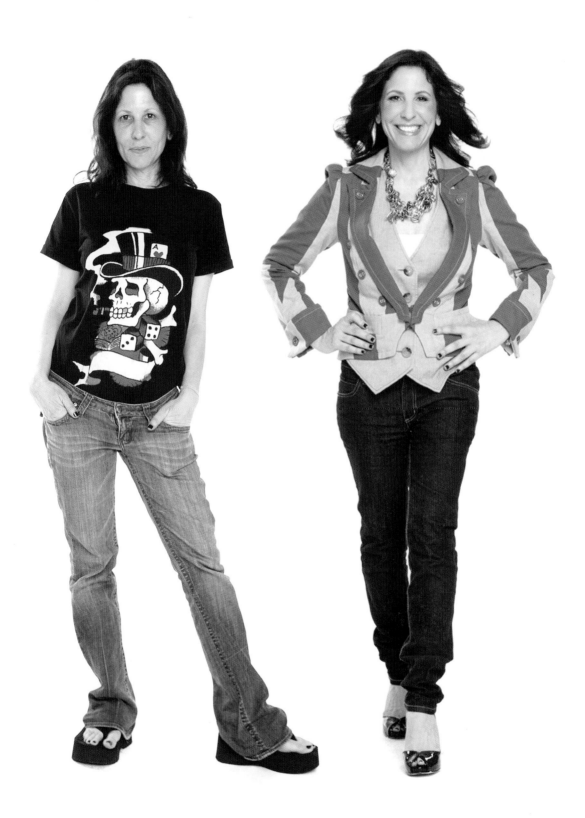

LORI

Darrell: Lori had very long, coarse hair, and there wasn't any particular style to it. She's a singer-songwriter, rock-and-roll chick, so I wanted to give her more of an edgy look. But Lori is also an actress, so we needed to keep it safe for auditions. My friend Sam Jacobson, an amazing colorist, colored her roots to give them a brighter brown tone, and did highlights to give her hair a glow and play better off of her fair complexion. Then I cut almost six inches of length off her hair, which must have been liberating for her. I gave her tons of layers to remove more weight. To finish, I blew it out with a smoothing serum and a big round boar-bristle brush. The result is fabulous, shiny, beautiful hair with tons of versatility.

Spencer: Lori is a total sweetheart, so I wanted to bring out the softer, feminine side of her to contrast with the sophisticated edge of Nick's styling. First I wanted to brighten and define the eye area: Lori's beautiful eyes got lost because her brows were so light. By adding shape and definition, it made a world of difference and balanced her face. Lori's eyes are deeper set, so I wanted to pull them forward. I started with the lash line and blended a soft taupe shadow to define the eyes, and added a pale shimmery shadow to reflect light. Her skin was really lovely and hydrated (great job, Kate!), so I didn't need to do much, just enhance what she had. I used very little foundation, mainly concealer around the eyes to soften dark circles, and a beige pink on the apples of her cheeks. We finished with a fleshy, nude lip, and Lori was ready to rock!

Nick: My goal with Lori was to bring out the glam in her glam-rock persona. She has such a tiny figure, but she wasn't showing it off *at all!* In fact, she was hiding under clothes that were two sizes too big. I especially wanted to give Lori's outfit different layers and texture. With this fabulous jacket, I gave her very strong and defined shoulders while keeping it simple and streamlined on the bottom. She is definitely rockin' in this outfit! We kept the attitude, but added a bit of chic sophistication.

Outfit:
- Marc by Marc Jacobs jacket and denim vest
- H&M white tank top
- Marc Jacobs Collection safety pin and crystal necklace
- Diane von Furstenberg black patent leather peep-toe heels
- Lori's own skinny jeans

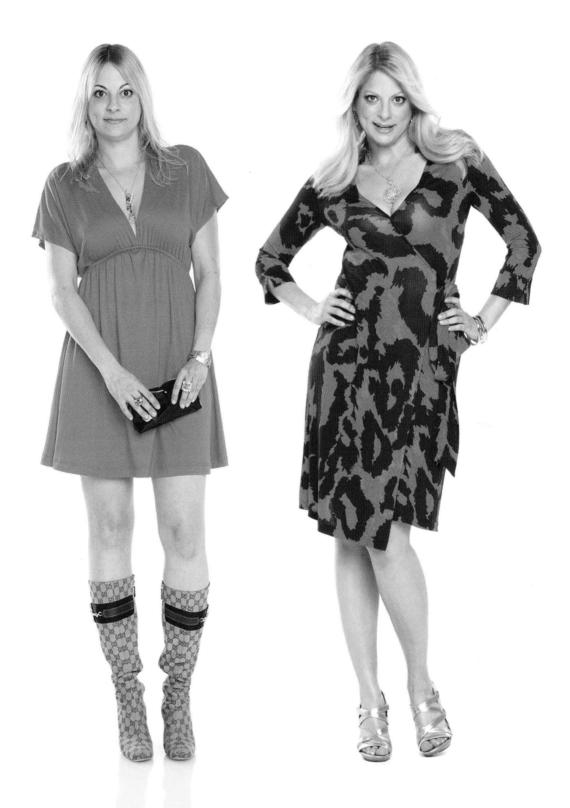

SHAYNE

Darrell: Shayne came to us with superfine, self-dyed blonde hair. Sam corrected her color by alternating platinum highlights with darker taupe lowlights. We wanted to add depth and dimension to her hair and make it appear thicker, so after the color work, I cut and layered it for added volume and lift. Once the color and cut were perfected, I styled Shayne's hair with a volumizer to give her a full, sexy, windblown movie-star look.

Spencer: Shayne might know a lot about people, but *I* could read *her* mind! I knew that there was a little sex kitten inside her sweet exterior, and I wanted to bring it out.

Shayne's eyes were a standout feature, but her brows were really dark and overpowered her face. I wanted to shift the focus back to her gorgeous brown eyes. So Darrell helped me lift her brows a few shades using hair color. Then, by adding a few individual flare lashes toward the outer third of her eyes, I was able to extend and elongate them, resulting in a sexy, doe-eyed shape. I opted for smoldering eyeliner in a silvery charcoal, smudged in a pinkish taupe, and highlighted her inner corners with a shimmering pale golden pink. The fresh, peach/pink blush I used brought life to her skin, balanced her eyes, and emphasized that bone structure. To finish, I dusted a sparkling bronzer across her décolletage to transition her face and neck into her body, adding glamour and glow. Just watch her purr!

Nick: Shayne may be a psychic by day, but I wanted to turn her into a glammed-up goddess for night! With the help of *my* inner fashion/psychic abilities, I somehow knew that she'd look divine in a boldly printed wrap dress. Shayne is tall and shapely, and this dress showed off her outstanding figure. It cinched her waist, framed her gorgeous face, and gave her a complete and put-together look, all in one garment. I predict that Shayne's fashion future is looking very bright—and sexy.

Outfit:
- Diane von Furstenberg jersey dress
- Diane von Furstenberg gold leather strappy heels
- Jessica Elliot necklace, earrings, and gold cuff bracelet

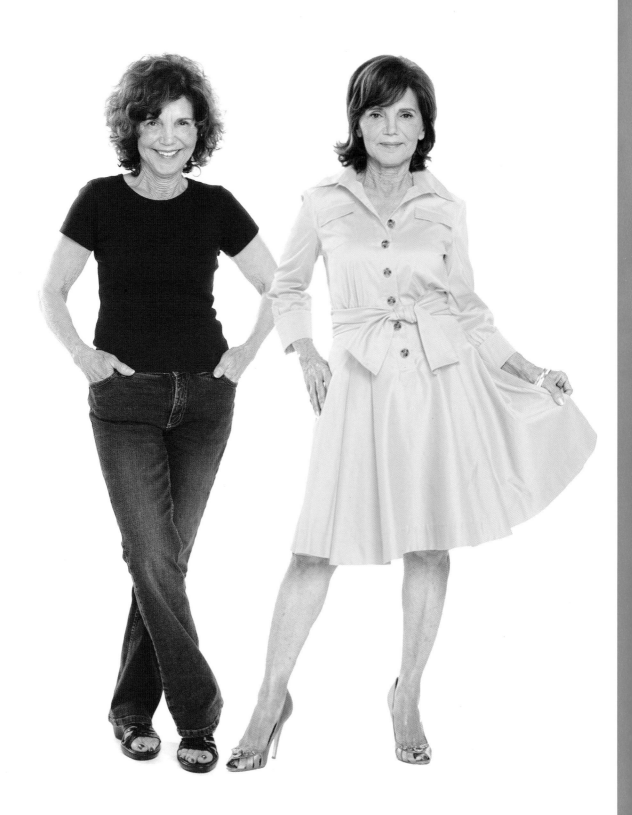

FAY

Darrell: I adore Fay. She came to me with a "bubble cut," and the color was uneven and needed a little boost of uniform highlights. Sam highlighted her hair evenly, and I cut the inner weight of her old style out. This created more layers and less round bulk. Fay is petite, and I wanted to create more height in her look, so creating a more vertical line in the haircut made her look taller—I also gave her a side part to help with that. Finally, I used a volumizer and round brush to give her a more youthful, trendy look. *Voilà!* She looks amazing now.

Spencer: What a gorgeous woman, who has learned to enjoy all the best that life has to offer. Right away, I knew that I could accentuate Fay's delicious personality with a splash of color. I started by complementing her chocolate eyes with a sweep of powdery lavender across her lids, and intensified the color with a deeper aubergine on the upper lash line. I used a burgundy mascara to keep her lashes natural looking and complement her eye-color palette. The finished look partnered her sophisticated sensibility with a timeless element of youthfulness. The result is a fun, subtle, and wearable combination. I also popped the apples of Fay's cheeks using a cool, fleshy pink. I chose a warmer, rose pink cream lipstick, with a light glaze of gloss on her pout. I created her makeup to be as sunny as that golden dress and sunshiny attitude. Fay perfectly shows that experimenting with color is not just for kids!

Nick: I knew there was a diva in Fay from the minute I met her, and that's what I wanted to bring out. With someone this petite, you have to be careful not to overwhelm her with clothes. I chose this simple belted shirtdress because it was the perfect color and silhouette for her frame, as well as the ideal length (right at the knee). Fay is ready for her red-carpet moment now, whether it's having tea with her girlfriends or just sipping a mint julep with me!

Outfit:
- Diane von Furstenberg cotton mustard yellow shirtdress
- Badgley Mischka gold heels
- H&M bracelets

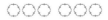

Afterword

Our skin, like life, is a work in progress. And as with almost anything that's worth doing, practice and attention make perfect. The road to complexion perfection may be paved for some and bumpy for others, but those who persevere will reach their goal.

It's important to understand that oftentimes along the way, you're going to reach a plateau. Maybe it's with your breakouts or your melasma, but things just don't seem to be getting any better, and you'll become frustrated. Just know that with patience and a little faith, you *will* get there. Andrew, the young singer you met in Chapter 10, was one of these cases—it took almost a year to get him entirely clear, but the payoff was amazing. To this day, I cry when I think of him. I'm so proud of the work we did and of his commitment and transformation. He has a joyful spirit, and now that his skin is clear, that joy is visible both inside and out. That young man absolutely lights up a room. So you have to work through the plateaus because you definitely will break through. Olympic athletes will tell you this. Successful actors will tell you this. It's no different with skin—I've witnessed it so many times.

So start now, whether you picked up this book because you have a healthy complexion and want to keep it that way, or because you were looking for guidance and solutions for some skin issue that's been bothering you. Begin with something simple, something you can work into your daily life. But don't delay. Think of a building: If it's kept up and cleaned regularly, it will age gracefully and possess the beauty, charm, and character that only age and experience can bring. And while it *can* be restored after years of neglect, it will take more work, time, and dedication.

There's no time like the present to get going. Have a facial. Invest in an eye cream. Drink more water. If you don't exfoliate—start. If you're breaking out—make a few changes in your diet. Honor yourself and your skin. After all, your complexion is constantly at work for you 24 hours a day, 7 days a week, 365 days a year. When you give back to it, you give back to yourself.

Challenge yourself and your self-concept. Many of the clients we made over for this book were nervous when we started. Maybe they weren't happy with their skin or how they'd aged, but they weren't really doing anything about their discontent. Yet every makeover client who walked into that photo studio for his or her "after" shot *glowed*. There was something you won't see in the photos—something different in the way these men and women carried themselves, in their step and in their eyes.

So make the time to take care of yourself, to enjoy who you are and your individual beauty. If you don't like something, find a way to fall in love with it or do something about it. Take control of who you are. Remember, you're in charge, so be the person you want to be. I truly believe that almost anything is possible in life, and believe it or not, it's my career in skin care that taught me this. So don't throw the towel in just yet—or ever. As a matter of fact, *grab* that towel. Cleanse your skin and begin to protect, hydrate, feed, stimulate, and detoxify your way to health and beauty. Because the path to complexion perfection leads to more than just glowing skin; it will lead to a happier, better *you.*

If I have one last message, it's about finding balance. Life is a journey that's meant to be savored. So celebrate your successes, big and small, and learn from your failures, for they're only lessons in disguise. Go after what you want; chase your dreams. Throw caution to the wind and listen to your heart. *Be fearless.* After all, that's the approach that led me here.

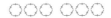

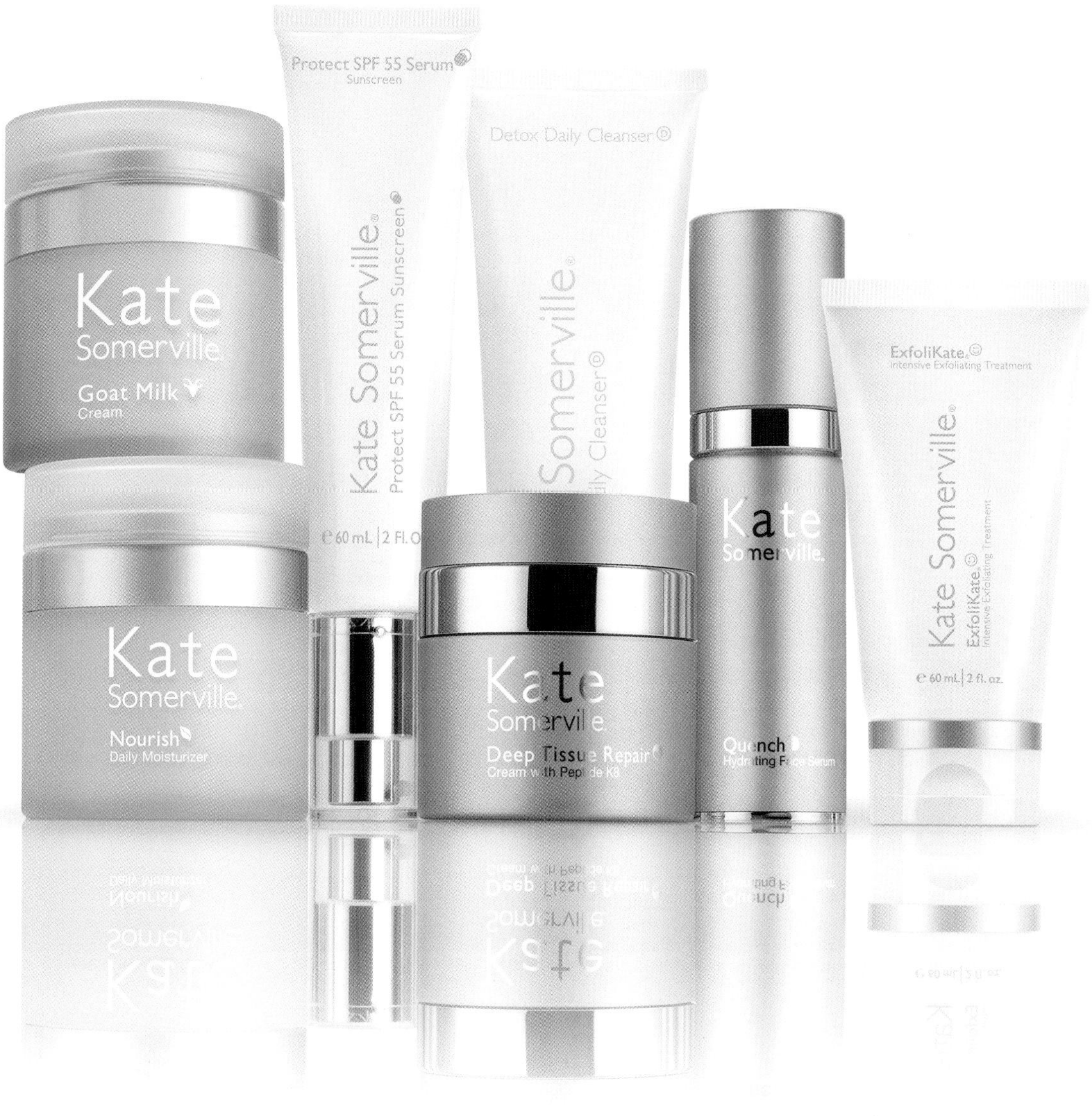
Protect SPF 55 Serum
Sunscreen
Kate Somerville
Protect SPF 55 Serum Sunscreen
60 mL | 2 Fl. O
Detox Daily Cleanser
Somerville
ily Cleanser
Kate
Somerville
Goat Milk
Cream
Kate
Somerville
Nourish
Daily Moisturizer
Kate
Somerville
Deep Tissue Repair
Cream with Peptide K8
Kate
Somerville
Quench
Hydrating Face Serum
ExfoliKate
Intensive Exfoliating Treatment
Kate Somerville
ExfoliKate
Intensive Exfoliating Treatment
60 mL | 2 fl. oz.

My Products

My products are my tools. Just like a
carpenter needs a hammer and some nails,
I need certain things to get the job done.
I started my own line because I was constantly wishing that the

product I was using had "just a little more glycolic" or a "more

powerful lightening agent." Then I met a chemist at a dermatology

meeting, and when I told him what I wanted to do, he began

compounding products for me. And that's how it all began.

My products don't make it onto the shelves until my clients have tried them and proven that they work. If they don't, we reformulate until they do! Now my line is sold in department stores and spas, on QVC, on the Internet, and at my clinic in Los Angeles.

Keep in mind that when you go to check out my products, you first need to type your skin as we did in Chapter 5, and then you can choose the appropriate ones for you.

Cleansers

Gentle Daily Wash is the perfect anti-aging cleanser, and great for dry skin and sensitive types. It's sulfate free.

Purify Exfoliating Cleanser. If you are really oily or have semi-acne-prone skin with lots of blackheads, you can use this gel cleanser. It's not great for dry skin types or those with delicate skin.

Detox Daily Cleanser is our most popular cleanser for acne. It contains calming B vitamins and won't overstrip the skin.

Exfoliators

ExfoliKate® Intensive Exfoliating Treatment has been touted by the press as "the next best thing" to seeing me in my clinic! Fruit enzymes dissolve dead skin cells, round microbeads buff them off of the surface, and lactic and salicylic acids further dissolve dead cells and work to lighten discoloration.

ExfoliKate® Gentle Intensive Exfoliating Treatment uses the same combination of technologies, gentle acids, fruit enzymes, and microbeads, but it's less intense.

Micro Glycolic Polisher is a professional-strength peel we've used for years in our facials at the clinic. It has 15 percent glycolic acid but is still formulated to be gentle.

Micro Lactic Polisher. For those with thin, sensitive skin, I recommend this. It encourages cell turnover and nicely prepares your skin for serums and moisturizers.

Toner

Clarifying Treatment Toner is alcohol free and has a base of witch hazel. But it also delivers phytic acid and Seb-control, an ingredient that tells the sebum gland to reduce oil production.

Treatments

Quench Hydrating Face Serum delivers lipids to plump up the skin cells and lock in moisture. It also has an advanced form of vitamin A to aid cell turnover.

Total Vitamin® Antioxidant Complex is a cocktail of vitamins that the skin needs to fight free radicals: B vitamins reduce general skin stress; vitamin C brightens; and vitamin E, green-tea extract, and other botanicals nourish the skin.

HydraKate Line Release™ Face Serum has peptides, amino acids, and hyaluronic acid to give you immediate tightening effects, hydration, and reduce wrinkles.

Anti Bac® Clearing Lotion boasts a unique formulation of encapsulated, timed-release benzoyl peroxide, so it gives your body little doses of it over time, not a huge blast all at once. This keeps the benzoyl peroxide from drying the skin out too much or creating sensitivity, which is almost always associated with the use of this ingredient.

EradiKate™ is "on the spot" relief for breakouts. When dabbed on as soon as pimples occur, it acts quickly to calm them and prevent further breakouts.

Moisturizers

Deep Tissue Repair Cream is my high-performance dream cream, with eight different wrinkle-fighting ingredients including Peptide K8, which is a powerful complex my chemist developed. This product builds collagen, restores elastin, and is clinically proven to reduce redness. So it's an antiwrinkle cream, yet it's calming.

Nourish Daily Moisture. This is a great cream for day or night because it feels light and contains the peptide compound Matrixyl 3000, which fights wrinkles. This moisturizer has vitamin A for cellular turnover as well, but is lighter than Deep Tissue Repair.

Goat Milk Cream has five ingredients, including proteins and amino acids, which come straight from goat's milk. It's nutritious and soothing to the skin and is amazing for dryness relief. It's actually a heavier moisturizer than Nourish, but is great for sensitive skin.

Oil Free Moisturizer. The sea-plant extracts in this product strengthen collagen and elastin and cause an immediate tightening. This moisturizer delivers hydration without using oils that can create congestion. It's also nice and lightweight, so anyone can use it.

Line Release® Under Eye Repair Cream. This light but effective product has state-of-the art ingredients including Matrixyl 3000 and Argireline.

Masks

Clearing Mask is for those with acne or oily skin to help heal breakouts and prevent further ones.

Mineral Mud Mask contains natural black silt that is perfect for every skin type. It calms, balances, adds hydration, and purifies the complexion.

Quench Hydrating Mask is an incredibly soothing and hydrating mask that restores water and moisture to the complexion.

Sun Protection

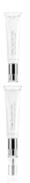

Protect SPF 30 Sunscreen. I developed this formula to protect all skin. It has antioxidants, in addition to broad-spectrum UVA and UVB protection.

Protect SPF 55 Serum Sunscreen is a broad-spectrum sunscreen that uses a combination of chemical and physical blocks to protect the skin. This advanced formulation is oil free and rich in antioxidants. It's ideal for every-day use, and works well under makeup.

Body

Goat Milk Body Lotion. The naturally occurring lactic acid in this product gently helps turn skin cells over, while the amino acids and proteins from the milk support the overall health of the skin.

Somer360° Tanning Towelettes. These are simple-to-use, streak-free tanning towels that give your body a golden (not orangey) glow. This paraben-free formula delivers that beautiful color, without the damage associated with tanning.

ExfoliKate® Body Intensive Exfoliating Treatment uses enzymes, acids, and beads to get rid of dead skin cells and polish and perfect.

At-Home Device

DermaLucent™ Handheld brings my clinic to *you!* It combines red LED and microcurrent to tighten, brighten, lift, and firm your complexion.

To learn more about my products and how I use them, please visit:
www.katesomerville.com.

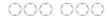

Thank You!

This project was a team effort, and I have so many people to thank. Most important are my son and husband: I love you so much and know how lucky I am. Thank you for the encouragement and understanding (as this took up some "family time"), and for always supporting my passion.

Thanks to Hay House for believing in me and that I had something valuable to share. Reid Tracy, you are so kind and supportive of your authors; it's been more than a pleasure to work with you. To Tracy O'Connor, who has helped me so much throughout the years and articulated my past, present, and future for this book—you are a beautiful and talented lady. Big thanks to Angela Hynes, who helped put my skin-care journey into words. Teri Laursen, your gorgeous design work brought beauty and life to this book!

Thank you to my teammates, the Skin Health Experts and front-desk angels at Kate Somerville, for the time and love you gave working on our "book" clients: what amazing results in just ten weeks! A special thanks to Melissa Haloossim for helping spearhead their treatment program, and to Rachita Patel and Francesca Alfano for your commitment to the cause. Thanks, too, to all of our Transformation clients.

Tremendous gratitude goes to photographers Jim Jordan and Jeff Xander for dedicating your time, talent, team, and heart to this project. Your karma just went up a notch! Thanks to Bryce and Jason Wheeler for the hard work, smiles, and graphics support. The amazing Glam Squad—Spencer Barnes, Nick Verreos, and Darrell Redleaf—you're the Indian chiefs of beauty. And thanks to all those who contributed to the shoot: Emese Szenasy of DVF; John Wade of Marc Jacobs; Teresa Kanode of Charles David; Nigel Dare of Nigel's Beauty Emporium; and Jessica Elliot, Shana Honeyman, Rachel Pally, Sam Jacobson, and David Paul for your expertise. Mike Ruiz—you are not only gorgeous, but generous.

Thanks to my friends and colleagues for sharing their knowledge, so I could pass it on in this book. Dr. David Rahm and your prettier half, Yvette La-Garde: you're inspirational. Thanks to Liz Mazurski for your warmth and years of support; as well as to chemists Fred Khoury, Jim Wilmot, John Garruto, and Dr. Bob Saute. Thanks to Cutera for creating safe and effective technologies, and to Wendy Oseas and Laura Cunningham. Blue Motion Studios, you have my appreciation for the illustrations. Ken Browning, you created this incredible opportunity. And thank you, Diamond Dave Somerville, for sharing your powerful and inspiring story.

Thank you to my family of makeup artists and hairstylists who have supported my team and me: David Gardner, Jeffrey Paul, Jake Bailey, Julie Hewitt, Monika Blunder, and Carola Gonzales. Tiffani Graves, I appreciate all of your styling support and would not look like this without you. Thank you to Martha Kramer for giving me *wings,* and to Jennifer Haliday and Dennis Lumpkin for all of your love since the beginning. Thanks to: Dawn Ahern, for organizing my busy life; Megan DeLoreto, for all of the extra help; JH Partners, for the space and support to do this project; Kyoko Getz, my soul-mate product developer; and Jon Bilock, for being "me" and holding down the fort. Brady Heyborne—thank you! A big hug to Marsha and Glen O'Connor for the proofreading. And thank you to QVC, Neiman Marcus, Nordstrom, Space NK, and Sephora for allowing me to educate others about, and help them with, their skin.

Special thanks to the talented celebrities who continue to support me and trust me with their faces: Julia Louis-Dreyfus, Felicity Huffman, Kerry Washington, Debra Messing, Kate Walsh, Paris Hilton, and Jennifer Coolidge. Immense gratitude to the beautiful Lisa Rinna for everything!

Tremendous thanks to everyone who supports me, my products, and my brand: I love you all.

Finally, thank you to my dad, my mom, and God for giving me life and guiding this journey.

About the Author

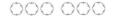

Kate Somerville is a widely respected paramedical esthetician with more than 18 years of experience in clinical skin care. She is the CEO and founder of Kate Somerville Skin Care and has a flourishing medi-skin clinic in Los Angeles. *People* magazine coined Kate the "A-list Beauty Guru," while *Allure* called her "Hollywood's Hottest Facialist." She has appeared on television shows including *Good Morning America, Dr. Phil,* and *Access Hollywood.* Kate's personal and professional experience served as her guiding principle when she developed her unique Skin Health Pyramid, a simple and strategic guide to achieving healthy, radiant skin. Her skin-care collection is distributed by leading retailers, luxury spas, and in doctors' offices, both domestically and abroad.

Website: **www.katesomerville.com**

Hay House Titles of Related Interest

YOU CAN HEAL YOUR LIFE, the movie, starring Louise L. Hay & Friends
(available as a 1-DVD program and an expanded 2-DVD set)
Watch the trailer at: **www.LouiseHayMovie.com**

THE SHIFT, the movie,
starring Dr. Wayne W. Dyer
(available as a 1-DVD program and an expanded 2-DVD set)
Watch the trailer at: **www.DyerMovie.com**

THE AGE OF MIRACLES: Embracing the New Midlife, by Marianne Williamson

THE ART OF EXTREME SELF-CARE: Transform Your Life One Month at a Time,
by Cheryl Richardson

*THE BEAUTY QUOTIENT FORMULA: How to Find Your Own Beauty Quotient to Look Your Best—
No Matter What Your Age,* by Robert Tornambe, M.D. (available April 2010)

*THE BODY KNOWS . . . HOW TO STAY YOUNG:
Healthy-Aging Secrets from a Medical Intuitive,* by Caroline Sutherland

FACE IT: What Women Really Feel as Their Looks Change,
by Vivian Diller, Ph.D., with Jill Muir-Sukenick, Ph.D., and Michele Willens

*THE HERBAL DETOX PLAN:
The Revolutionary Way to Cleanse and Revive Your Body,* by Xandria Williams

HOME SPA: Creating Your Own Spa Experience with Aromatherapy, by Judith White

SECRETS & MYSTERIES: The Glory and Pleasure of Being a Woman, by Denise Linn

TRANSCENDENT BEAUTY: It Begins with a Single Choice . . . to Be! by Crystal Andrus

YOUR BEST FACE: Looking Your Best Without Plastic Surgery,
by Brandith Irwin, M.D., and Mark McPherson, Ph.D.

All of the above are available at your local bookstore, or may be ordered by visiting:
Hay House USA: **www.hayhouse.com**®; Hay House Australia: **www.hayhouse.com.au;**
Hay House UK: **www.hayhouse.co.uk;** Hay House South Africa: **www.hayhouse.co.za;**
Hay House India: **www.hayhouse.co.in**

We hope you enjoyed this Hay House book.
If you'd like to receive our online catalog featuring additional information on
Hay House books and products, or if you'd like to find out more about the
Hay Foundation, please contact:

Hay House, Inc.
P.O. Box 5100
Carlsbad, CA 92018-5100

(760) 431-7695 or **(800) 654-5126**
(760) 431-6948 (fax) or **(800) 650-5115 (fax)**
www.hayhouse.com® • **www.hayfoundation.org**

Published and distributed in Australia by:
Hay House Australia Pty. Ltd., 18/36 Ralph St., Alexandria NSW 2015
Phone: 612-9669-4299 • *Fax:* 612-9669-4144 • www.hayhouse.com.au

Published and distributed in the United Kingdom by:
Hay House UK, Ltd., 292B Kensal Rd., London W10 5BE
Phone: 44-20-8962-1230 • *Fax:* 44-20-8962-1239 • www.hayhouse.co.uk

Published and distributed in the Republic of South Africa by:
Hay House SA (Pty), Ltd., P.O. Box 990, Witkoppen 2068
Phone/Fax: 27-11-467-8904 • info@hayhouse.co.za • www.hayhouse.co.za

Published in India by: Hay House Publishers India,
Muskaan Complex, Plot No. 3, B-2, Vasant Kunj, New Delhi 110 070
Phone: 91-11-4176-1620 • *Fax:* 91-11-4176-1630 • www.hayhouse.co.in

Distributed in Canada by: Raincoast, 9050 Shaughnessy St., Vancouver, B.C. V6P 6E5
Phone: (604) 323-7100 • *Fax:* (604) 323-2600 • www.raincoast.com

<u>**Take Your Soul on a Vacation**</u>

Visit **www.HealYourLife.com**® to regroup, recharge, and reconnect with your own magnificence.
Featuring blogs, mind-body-spirit news, and life-changing wisdom from Louise Hay and friends.

Visit **www.HealYourLife.com** today!

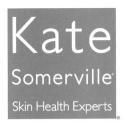

Kate Somerville®
Skin Health Experts®

A SPECIAL GIFT FOR READERS OF

Complexion Perfection!

10% off
and Free Shipping

on your first purchase of Kate Somerville Skin Care!

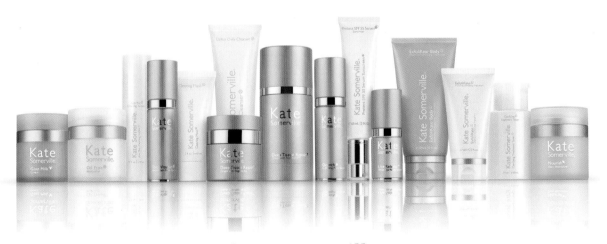

www.katesomerville.com

Call or log on today and provide Promo Code: KATEBOOK

Mind Your Body,
Mend Your Spirit

Hay House is the ultimate resource for inspirational and health-conscious books, audio programs, movies, events, e-newsletters, member communities, and much more.

Visit **www.hayhouse.com®** today and nourish your soul.

UPLIFTING EVENTS

Join your favorite authors at live events in a city near you or log on to **www.hayhouse.com** to visit with Hay House authors online during live, interactive Web events.

INSPIRATIONAL RADIO

Daily inspiration while you're at work or at home. Enjoy radio programs featuring your favorite authors, streaming live on the Internet 24/7 at **HayHouseRadio.com®**. Tune in and tune up your spirit!

VIP STATUS

Join the Hay House VIP membership program today and enjoy exclusive discounts on books, CDs, calendars, card decks, and more. You'll also receive 10% off all event reservations (excluding cruises). Visit **www.hayhouse.com/wisdom** to join the Hay House Wisdom Community™.

Visit **www.hayhouse.com** and enter priority code 2723
during checkout for special savings!
(One coupon per customer.)

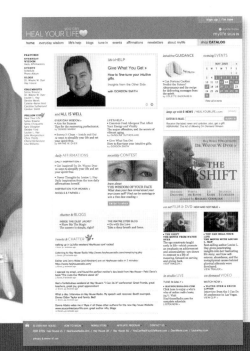